Paleo Italian

Slow Cooking

Over 150 Authentic Italian Recipes for the Electric Slow Cooker

Dominique DeVito

with Breea Johnson, M.S., R.D., L.D.N.

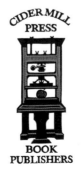

CIDER MILL PRESS

BOOK PUBLISHERS

Kennebunkport, Maine

13-Digit ISBN: 978-1604334647
10-Digit ISBN: 1-60433-464-9

This book may be ordered by mail from the publisher. Please include $4.95 for postage and handling.
Please support your local bookseller first!

Books published by Cider Mill Press Book Publishers are available at special discounts for bulk purchases in the United States by corporations, institutions, and other organizations. For more information, please contact the publisher.

Cider Mill Press Book Publishers
"Where good books are ready for press"
12 Spring Street
PO Box 454
Kennebunkport, Maine 04046

Visit us on the web!
www.cidermillpress.com

Design by Alicia Freile, Tango Media
Typeset by Gwen Galeone, Tango Media
Typography: Archer, Chaparral Pro, Helvetica Neue and Voluta
All images used under license from Shutterstock.com.
Printed in China

1 2 3 4 5 6 7 8 9 0
First Edition

Paleo Italian

Slow Cooking

Contents

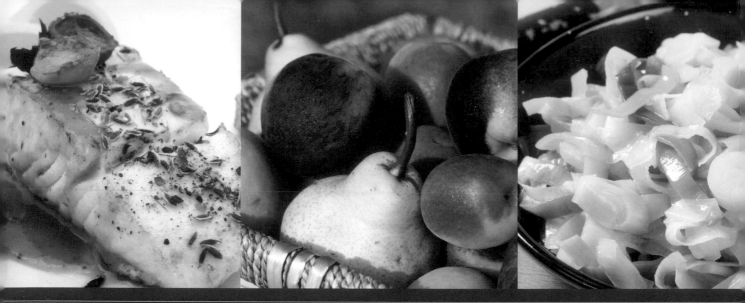

Introduction

What Is the Paleo Diet, and Why Is It Good for Me?

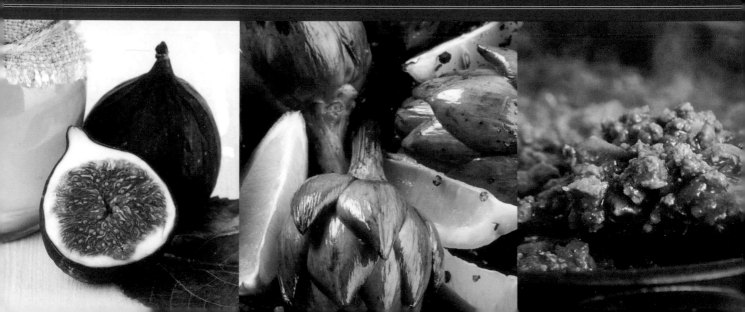

*F*irst, congratulations on your interest in Paleo eating. Going Paleo is more than just diet, though it certainly starts there. It's also about making choices for a healthier lifestyle all around. And that's wonderful.

Like any bold change you want to make to better your health, however, this one will require some sacrifices and will take some adjustment. This may sound discouraging, but it's important to be honest. The Paleo plan requires that you give up foods that you may have learned to associate with comfort and good times, like sugar, white bread and potatoes, processed foods, and dairy. I know, it sounds scary. The good news—and it's really good news!—is that the sacrifices you'll make have huge payoffs for your health.

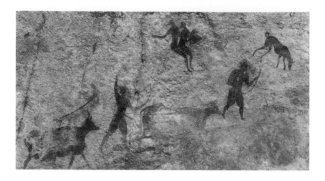

If you're like me, within the first few weeks of making the change to the Paleo diet, you should experience:

* Increased energy
* Moderate weight loss
* Improved digestion
* Improved skin tone and hair condition
* Improved mood, including more restful sleep

If these are the benefits you're seeking, you won't be disappointed. The added bonus of this book is that you'll learn to use the slow cooker to keep you on the Paleo diet, so you'll have a collection of recipes that will make eating—and enjoying meals—easy and affordable at the same time you'll be reaping the benefits of Paleo.

What Is Paleo?

"Paleo" is short for *Paleolithic*. This was the time period dating from approximately 2 million to 12,000 BCE. Next was the Mesolithic Era, from roughly 12,000 to 8,000 BCE, and the Neolithic Era, or roughly 8,000 to 5,000 BCE and the transition to a more agricultural, domestic lifestyle for ancient humans. The Paleolithic era is also referred to as the Stone Age. It is when our ancestors became much more skilled at hunting with stone tools, which enabled them to hunt animals more effectively. For most of this period, humans were simple hunter-gatherers, competing for food sources with the likes of wooly mammoths and savage wooly rhinoceroces, giant deer, bison, musk ox, hare, and others. They were much more in synch with their environments—out of necessity—and adapted to the demands of the day, spending many hours foraging and hunting.

Because caves afforded some of the best protection against the wildlife and the elements, we have come to refer to our ancestors of these eras as "cavemen," and thus the Paleo(lithic) diet is sometimes referred to as the *caveman diet*. It is a simplification, of course, but it also provides a great concept for the diet, which is one based largely on meat, fish, eggs, vegetables, and fruits. It's also a fitting concept for the lifestyle of Paleo people—on the move, ever watchful, keenly aware of their surroundings.

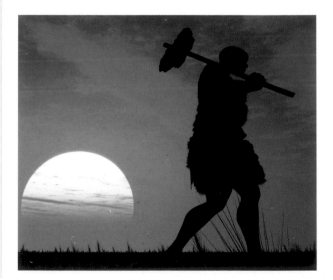

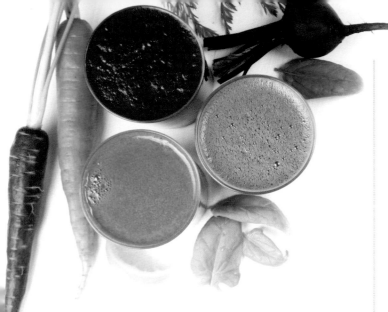

Paleo for the Modern World

Though we may be borrowing from the concept of "necessity" eating and activity from our Paleo brethren (and sistren), be glad we are living in today's modern world where this is, for us, a choice rather than a necessity. If we had to get out there and bring down our meals on a regular basis, we wouldn't have time to read—or write—cookbooks such as these! We've come a long way, baby—for real!—and there's no need to go backward. That's another great thing about today's Paleo diet (and this cookbook): It contains far more variety than a caveperson could have ever conceived of, and healthier means of preparation, as well!

Another consideration for the modern Paleo is the very real awareness of the impact of domesticated meat production on the planet. Cavemen weren't killing herds of black Angus beef cattle; they were taking on animals in the wild. And the caveman population wasn't at nearly 7 billion worldwide. If everyone went Paleo, the increased demand for domesticated meat could do more harm than good on a global level.

These are discussion points beyond the scope of this cookbook, but ones that Paleo enthusiasts debate frequently, and rightly so. As the benefits of the diet to their overall health make them even greater supporters of it, they explore more and more of its aspects. One of the founding fathers of the Paleo diet and lifestyle is Loren Cordain, PhD. He is the author of *The Paleo Diet* and several spinoffs from that book. He speaks about the diet around the world. He has a website (www.the paleodiet.com) and a blog and is considered "the leading expert on paleolithic diets and founder of the paleo movement." He is an excellent resource to tap into as you learn more about Paleo.

And now, let's eat!

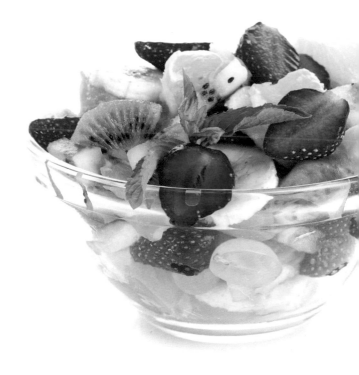

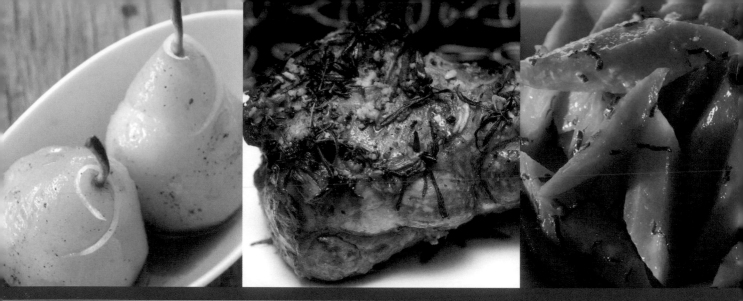

Chapter 1

The Italian Kitchen Goes Paleo

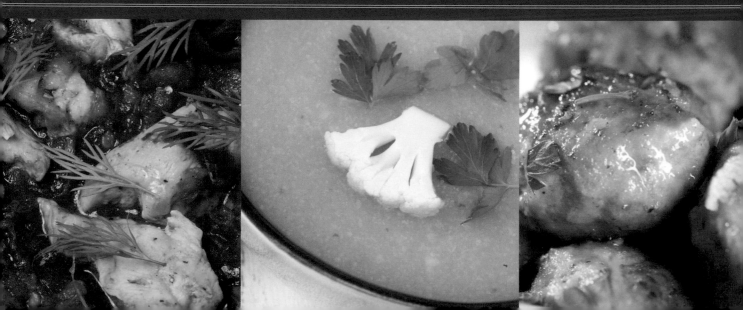

This is the part of going Paleo where the rubber meets the road, where your commitment will come smack up against your current eating habits. It's not that you won't be able to fill your pantry and fridge with a great selection of Paleo-friendly foods. It's just that in order to do that, you first need to eliminate the foods that aren't part of the Paleo diet. This chapter outlines what you want to remove from your pantry and what you want to stock up on.

Out Before In

So that you aren't distracted or tempted in misleading directions early on, you want to immediately clear out what you won't need or want from your cabinets. Find a sturdy cardboard box or some of your larger recyclable grocery bags. You want to pack up the intact packages of foods you won't be needing anymore and easily transport them to a family member, friend, or your local food pantry.

Start with your pantry. You want to remove any grains—rice of any kind, pasta, noodles, quinoa, oatmeal, etc. You'll also want to purge your shelves of any foods that include sugar. Read the labels if you're uncertain, as this includes any artificial sweeteners, as well, and there are many of them. Some of the more common are saccharine, aspartame, sucralose, corn syrup, and high fructose corn syrup. Next, remove any containers of processed oils—vegetable oil, canola oil, and peanut oil are some of the more popular. Anything that is hydrogenated or partially hydrogenated has to go. Don't worry; fats are a necessary part of a Paleo diet and good health, and there are several on the "must-have" list.

While vegetables are a major component of the Paleo diet, legumes are off limits, as they contain contribute to digestive distress and bloating. Legumes include most types of beans (kidney, garbanzo, pinto, fava, and soy). You may be surprised how many legumes you have in your pantry, as they are staples in soups, stews, and even salads. Fortunately, legumes that are more pod than pea can be included in the diet (more on those later).

Move on to your refrigerator and freezer. Say goodbye to dairy—milk, margarine, cheese, yogurt,

ice cream. Say goodbye to bottled salad dressings, deli meats, juices, and anything that contains nitrates, sweeteners, artificial ingredients, or other non-Paleo ingredients, as mentioned above. You can save your butter and turn it into ghee, which is clarified butter where the water and solids are cooked off so that only the butterfat remains.

To summarize, here's a list of foods and foodstuffs you need to remove from your home:

* Pastas and other grains
* Oatmeal
* Breakfast cereals
* Granola
* Rice
* Breads, crackers, chips
* Sugar, including brown, light brown, and confectioner's
* Artificial sweeteners and products that contain them
* Candy
* Cookies
* Vegetable oil
* Canola oil
* Peanut oil
* Sunflower oil
* Corn oil
* Soybean oil
* Shortening
* Peanut butter, mixed nuts (especially cocktail peanuts)
* Cans or bags of beans—red, kidney, pinto, lima, garbanzo
* Jams and jellies
* Salad dressings
* Soy sauce

* Packaged sauces or condiments, including ketchup and mustard
* Milk, butter, cream, margarine, yogurt, ice cream, and other dairy

Now heed this advice: Immediately take away the foods you've removed! You do not want to be tempted by any of them.

In and Begin

Once you've removed the no-no's, it's time to stock up on what will become the staples of your new, healthier diet. Besides referencing the lists here, browse through this cookbook and take note of ingredients that sound especially good. Remember, one of the main reasons that a Paleo diet can be so healthy for you is that it is focused on fresher, more easily digested food sources. When considering what to stock up on, always think fresh.

Be forewarned: Your body will go through cravings for foods you once took for granted—especially those with sugar—and you'll want to be sure you have the makings of something really tasty so you can feel good about your decision and stick with your commitment.

For the Cupboard

Most of your ancillary ingredients on the Paleo diet will be seasonings, as the essentials are truly simple: meat, fish, eggs, vegetables, fruits and berries. Depending on how old some of your current selections are, you may want to start over; that's up to you. Stock up on all of these so you have lots of options when it's time to cook. And while it's important to have a great selection of seasonings, remember that fresher is always better, so use fresh herbs when you can.

Stock up on:
* Dried herbs, including basil, parsley, oregano, chives, mint, thyme, tarragon, sage, bay leaves, and rosemary
* Ground spices, including cayenne pepper, cumin, coriander, ginger, nutmeg, clove, curry powder, all-spice, paprika, chili powder, mustard, and cardamom
* Pepper and iodized sea salt

There are all kinds of spice combinations on the market today, and almost all are fair game for Paleo cooking. Just be sure to read the ingredients and make sure they don't contain artificial sweeteners or preservatives.

Oils and Other Staples

Your pantry will look woefully bare without cans and jars and containers of beans, jams, cereals, pasta, spaghetti sauces, and snacks. Yikes! Time to move in what is Paleo-approved:
* Oils contribute necessary fats to a diet, and are essential for cooking. Those that can be used for a Paleo diet are extra-virgin olive oil, coconut oil (unrefined), avocado oil, nut oils (like walnut or almond), and seed oils (flax and sesame, for example).
* Dried fruits, which make for great snacks—in moderation and with no additional sweetener added
* Dry or roasted nuts, like almonds, walnuts, pistachios, and cashews. Again, in moderation.
* Broths and stocks, including chicken, beef and vegetable broths, so long as there are no sugars or soy in them
* Vinegars, including red wine, balsamic, apple cider and coconut
* Olives packed in water with minimal salt

* Pickles jarred without sugars or chemicals
* Canned fish packed in water or olive oil (not soybean oil), including tuna, salmon, and sardines
* Tomato paste and salsa without added sugar, corn, or wheat
* Fish sauce
* Hot sauce
* Mustard
* Coconut aminos (a soy-free seasoning sauce that's loaded with amino acids)
* Baking products: almond flour, baking powder, baking soda, cocoa powder, chocolate (75% cocoa and higher), honey, maple syrup, and arrowroot powder (a thickener)

Paleo and Fats

Oils and butter are sources of fat in cooking, and are both necessary. Paleo-appropriate oils are listed above, but you can also cook with other fats.

One of the sources of fat referenced often in this book is ghee. The source of ghee is butter, and butter is made from cow's milk (most typically), and dairy is an ingredient to be avoided on a Paleo diet. The reason ghee is acceptable is because it is butter that has had the most commonly found allergic dairy components—casein and lactose—removed. What's left is the pure butterfat. Added advantages of ghee are that it won't smoke at higher temperatures (regular butter can tolerate about 350 degrees; ghee can go to about 450 degrees) and that it stores well and stays fresh longer than butter.

You'll see references to the use of ghee throughout this book, and also to clarified butter. While some consider them synonymous, and in fact they are both the result of butter being slow heated so that the water evaporates and the solids remain, clarified

butter has the fats poured off during the cooking process to prevent browning and ghee doesn't. Letting the fats remain and browning somewhat yields a somewhat nutty and richer flavor to ghee than to clarified butter.

Other Paleo fats for cooking besides olive oil (at low temperatures) and coconut oil that can be used are red duck fat, lard, and tallow. They are far less common, though.

Protein Sources

These will comprise the bulk of the Paleo diet, so it's important to shop smart for what is healthiest. For meats like beef, lamb, and pork, you want to be sure you're purchasing grass-fed, organically raised sources. Poultry should be free-range. The best fish is wild-caught, and cold-water, oily fishes like herring, anchovies, mackerel, salmon, and sardines are the highest in omega-3 fatty acids.

The most economical way to stock up on meats and fish is to buy in bulk if possible. Find a farmer at a farmer's market whose meats meet with your approval, and talk to him or her about purchasing a side of an animal. It may be worth investing in a freezer to accommodate this quantity, but it is definitely more economical in the long run.

The Paleo diet includes high-quality sources of:
* Beef
* Pork
* Lamb
* Poultry
* Eggs
* Fish and seafood
* Game meats (pheasant, boar, bear, elk, etc.)

Remember, too, that organ meats (liver, kidneys, brain) were a true Paleo staple (and often the highest-prized cuts), so be sure to keep these in your freezer.

Vegetables

The only items you'll need to avoid in the produce section of your grocery store—or at the farmer's market—are corn, peas, and white potatoes. So whether your tastes run to leafy greens, crunchy carrots, zucchini, squashes, cabbage and Brussels sprouts, asparagus, beets, even artichokes—indulge in them and enjoy.

Fruits and Berries

As you transition to Paleo, if you've been used to ending your meals with a sweet treat, the sugar monster will haunt you. It will seem like everywhere you look there are sweet foods that you can't eat.

To help beat back the sugar monster, be sure you have fruits and berries with you at all times. Keep a small bag of dried fruit in the car or in your desk drawer. If you crave something soft and sweet, turn to a ripe banana. You can enjoy oranges, apples, tangerines, strawberries, raspberries, peaches, pineapples, grapes, melons, even watermelon.

Tutto Italiano

There are some ingredients that are synonymous with their country of origin. For example, one associates butter with French cooking; tomatoes with Italian cuisine; or curry with Indian food. When going Paleo Italiano, these are the (Paleo appropriate) ingredients you want to have in stock at all times, as they are staples of Italian cooking throughout Italy:

* Anchovies
* Balsamic vinegar
* Basil
* Bay leaves
* Broth
* Capers
* Garlic
* Marjoram
* Nutmeg
* Extra virgin olive oil
* Olives
* Oregano
* Pancetta
* Parsley (flat leaf)
* Black pepper
* Porcini mushrooms
* Prosciutto
* Radicchio
* Rosemary
* Sage
* Tomatoes
* Truffles
* Tuna

You can see from this list what Italian cuisine is all about: freshness of flavors. When you think about combining tomatoes, garlic, olive oil, and basil in Italy, you can imagine yourself in the Italian countryside where all has been sourced within 5 kilometers. You can do the same thing here in the United States if you live where these ingredients are grown locally. Or you can buy Italian pancetta and make an incredible omelet with it, using local eggs and flat-leaf parsley. Become familiar with the seasonings and versatility of these primary components, and Italy will come alive in your kitchen. *Delicioso!*

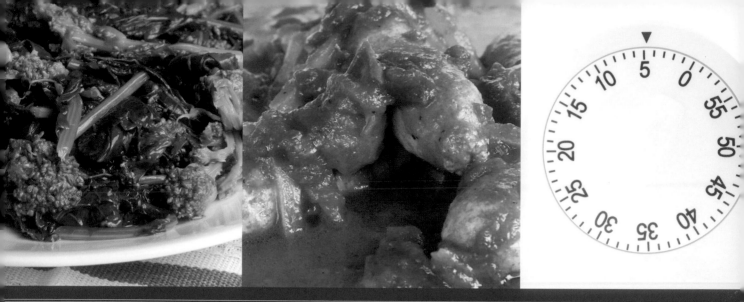

Chapter 2

Slowly Does It:

A Guide to Slow Cookers and the Wonders of Slow Cooking

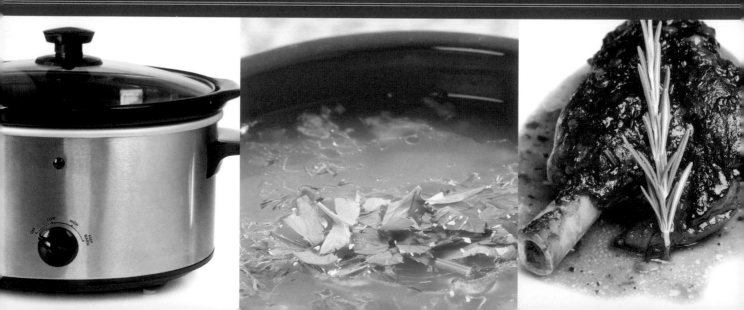

*L*uckily for all of us who are "science challenged," it doesn't take a degree in physics to operate a slow cooker. It's about the easiest machine there is on the market. It's certainly far less complicated than an espresso machine or even a waffle maker. In this chapter you'll learn about slow cookers and how to get the best results from them.

Slow cookers are inexpensive to operate; they use about as much electricity as a 60-watt bulb. They are also as easy to operate as flipping on a light switch.

Slow cookers operate by cooking food using indirect heat at a low temperature for an extended period of time. Here's the difference: Direct heat is the power of a stove burner underneath a pot, while indirect heat is the overall heat that surrounds foods as they bake in the oven.

You can purchase a slow cooker for as little as $20 at a discount store, while the top-of-the-line ones sell for more than $200. They all function in the same simple way; what increases the cost is the "bells and whistles" factors. Slow cookers come in both round and oval shapes, but they operate the same regardless of shape.

Food is assembled in a pottery insert that fits inside a metal housing and is topped with a clear lid. The food cooks from the heat generated by the circular heating wires encased between the slow cooker's outer and inner layers of metal. The coils never directly touch the crockery insert. As the element heats, it gently warms the air between the two layers of metal, and it is the hot air that touches the pottery. This construction method eliminates the need for stirring because no part of the pot gets hotter than any other.

On the front of this metal casing is the control knob. All slow cookers have Low and High settings, and most also have a Stay Warm position. Some new machines have a programmable option that enables you to start food on High and then the slow cooker automatically reduces the heat to Low after a programmed time.

The largest variation in slow cookers is their size, which range from tiny 1-quart models that are excellent for hot dips and fondue but fairly useless for anything else to gigantic 7-quart models that are excellent for large families and large batches.

Rival introduced the first slow cooker, the Crock-Pot, in 1971, and the introductory slogan remains true more than 35 years later: It "cooks all day while the cook's away." Like such trademarked names as Kleenex for paper tissue or Formica for plastic laminate, Crock-Pot has almost become synonymous with the slow cooker. However, not all slow cookers are Crock-Pots, so the generic term is used in this book.

Most of the recipes in this book were written for and tested in a 4- or 5-quart slow cooker; that is what is meant by *medium*. Either of those sizes makes enough for four to eight people, depending on the recipe.

Slow Cookers and Food Safety

Questions always arise as to the safety of slow cookers. The Food Safety and Inspection Service of the U.S. Department of Agriculture approves slow cooking as a method for safe food preparation. The lengthy cooking and the steam created within the tightly covered pot combine to destroy any bacteria that might be present in the food. But you do have to be careful.

It's far more common for food-borne illness to start with meat, poultry, and seafood than from contaminated fruits and vegetables. That is why it's not wise to cook whole chickens or cuts of meat larger than those specified in the recipes in this book because during slow cooking, these large items remain too long in the bacterial "danger zone"— between 40°F and 140°F. It is important that food reaches the higher temperature in less than two hours and remains at more than 140°F for at least 30 minutes.

Getting a jump-start on dinner while you're preparing breakfast may seem like a Herculean task, and it is possible to prep the ingredients destined for the slow cooker the night before—with some limitations. If you cut meat or vegetables in advance, store them separately in the refrigerator and layer them in the slow cooker in the morning. However, do not store the cooker insert in the refrigerator because that

> If you want to cook large roasts, brown them under the oven broiler or in a skillet on top of the stove over direct heat before you place them into the slow cooker. This will help the chilled meat heat up faster as well as produce a dish that is more visually appealing. Also, begin with liquid that is boiling.

will also increase the amount of time it takes to heat the food to a temperature that kills bacteria.

Concern about food safety extends to after a meal is cooked and the leftovers are ready for storage. As long as the temperature remains 140°F or higher, food will stay safe for many hours in the slow cooker. Leftovers, however, should never be refrigerated in the crockery insert because it will take them too long to go through the "danger zone" in the other direction—from hot to cold.

Freeze or refrigerate leftovers in shallow containers within two hours after a dish has finished cooking. Also, food should never be reheated in the slow cooker because it takes too long for chilled food to reheat. Bacteria are a problem on cooked food as well as raw ingredients. The slow cooker can be used to keep food warm—and without the fear of burning it—once it has been reheated on the stove or in the oven.

One of the other concerns about food safety and the slow cooker is if there is a loss of power in the house—especially if you don't know when it occurred in the cooking process. If you're home, and the amount of time was minimal, add it back into your end time. If the time without power increases to more than 30 minutes, finish the food by conven-

tional cooking, adding more liquid, if necessary. However, if you set the slow cooker before you left for work and realize from electric clocks that power was off for more than an hour, it's best to discard the food, even if it looks done. You have no idea if the power outage occurred before the food passed through the "danger zone." Better safe than sorry.

> Always thaw food before placing it in the slow cooker to ensure the trip from 40°F to 140°F is accomplished quickly and efficiently. Starting with a frozen pot roast or chicken breast will make it impossible for the Low temperature of the slow cooker to accomplish this task.

Slow Cooker Hints

Slow cookers can be perplexing if you're not accustomed to using one. Here are some general tips to help you master slow cooker conundrums:

* Remember that cooking times are wide approximations—within hours rather than minutes! That's because the age or power of a slow cooker as well as the temperature of ingredients must be taken into account. Check the food at the beginning of the stated cooking time, and then gauge whether it needs more time and about how much time. If carrots or cubes of potato are still rock-hard, for example, turn the heat to High if cooking on Low, and realize that you're looking at another hour or so.

* Foods cook faster on the bottom of a slow cooker than at the top because there are more

heat coils and they are totally immersed in the simmering liquid.

* Appliance manufacturers say that slow cookers can be left on either High or Low unattended, but use your own judgment. If you're going to be out of the house all day, it's advisable to cook food on Low. If, on the other hand, you're going to be gone for just a few hours, the food will be safe on High.

* If you want a sauce to have a more intense flavor, you can reduce the liquid in two ways. If cooking on Low, raise the heat to High, and remove the lid for the last hour of cooking. This will achieve some evaporation of the liquid. Or, remove the liquid either with a bulb baster or strain the liquid from the solids, and reduce them in a saucepan on the stove.

> Many families don't think to use their slow cookers in the summer. But running the slow cooker doesn't raise the kitchen temperature by even a degree, and you can be outside enjoying the warm weather while it's cooking away.

Slow Cooker Cautions

Slow cookers are benign, but they are electrical appliances with all the concomitant hazards of any machine plugged into a live wire. Be careful that the cord is not frayed in any way, and plug the slow cooker into an outlet that is not near the sink.

Here are some tips on how to handle them:

* Never leave a slow cooker plugged in when not in use. It's all too easy to accidentally turn it on and not notice until the crockery insert cracks from overheating with nothing in it.

* Conversely, do not preheat the empty insert while you're preparing the food because the insert could crack when you add the cold food.

* Never submerge the metal casing in water or fill it with water. The inside of the metal does occasionally get dirty, but you can clean it quite well with an abrasive cleaner and then wipe it with a damp cloth or paper towel. While it's not aesthetically pleasing to see dirty metal, food never touches it, so if there are a few drips here and there it's not really important.

* Always remember that the insert is fragile, so don't drop it. Also, don't put a hot insert on a cold counter; that could cause it to break, too. The reverse is also true. While you can use the insert as a casserole in a conventional oven (assuming the lid is glass and not plastic), it cannot be put into a preheated oven if chilled.

* Resist the temptation to look and stir. Every time you take the lid off the slow cooker, you need to add 10 minutes of cooking time if cooking on High and 20 minutes if cooking on Low to compensate. Certain recipes in this book instruct you to add ingredients during the cooking time. In those cases the heat loss from opening the pot has been factored in to the total cooking time.

* Don't add more liquid to a slow cooker recipe than that specified in the recipe. Even if the food is not submerged in liquid when you start, foods such as meats and vegetables give off liquid as they cook; in the slow cooker, that additional liquid does not evaporate.

High-Altitude Adjustment

Rules for slow cooking, along with all other modes of cooking, change when the slow cooker is located more than 3,000 feet above sea level. At high altitudes the air is thinner so water boils at a lower temperature and comes to a boil more quickly. The rule is to always cook on High when above 3,000 feet; use the Low setting as a Keep Warm setting.

Other compensations are to reduce the liquid in a recipe by a few tablespoons and add about 5 to 10 percent more cooking time. The liquid may be bubbling, but it's not 212°F at first.

Converting Recipes for the Slow Cooker

Once you feel comfortable with your slow cooker, you'll probably want to use it to prepare your favorite recipes you now cook on the stove or in the oven. The best recipes to convert are wet ones with a lot of liquid, such as stews, soups, chilies, and other braised foods. Not all dishes can be easily converted to slow cooked dishes. Even if a dish calls for liquid, if it's supposed to be cooked or baked uncovered, chances are it will not be successfully transformed to a slow cooker recipe, because the food will not brown and the liquid will not evaporate.

The easiest way to convert your recipes is to find a similar one in this book and use its cooking time for guidance. When looking for a similar recipe, take into account the amount of liquid specified as well as the quantity of food. The liquid transfers the heat from the walls of the insert into the food itself, and the liquid heats in direct proportion to its measure.

You should look for similar recipes as well as keep in mind some general guidelines:

* Most any stew or roast takes 8 to 12 hours on Low and 4 to 6 hours on High.
* Chicken dishes cook more rapidly. Count on 6 to 8 hours on Low and 3 to 4 hours on High.
* Quadruple the time from conventional cooking to cooking on Low, and at least double it for cooking on High.
* Cut back on the amount of liquid used in stews and other braised dishes by about half. Unlike cooking on the stove or in the oven, there is little to no evaporation in the slow cooker.
* For soups, cut back on the liquid by one-third if the soup is supposed to simmer uncovered, and cut back by one-fourth if the soup is simmered covered. Even when covered, a soup that is simmering on the stove has more evaporation than one cooked in the slow cooker.

Modern slow cookers heat slightly hotter than those made thirty years ago; the Low setting on a slow cooker is about 200°F while the High setting is close to 300°F. If you have a vintage appliance, it's a good idea to test it to make sure it still has the power to heat food sufficiently. Leave 2 quarts water at room temperature overnight, and then pour the water into the slow cooker in the morning. Heat it on Low for 8 hours. The temperature should be 185°F after 8 hours. Use an instant read thermometer to judge it. If it is lower, any food you cook in this cooker might not pass through the danger zone rapidly enough.

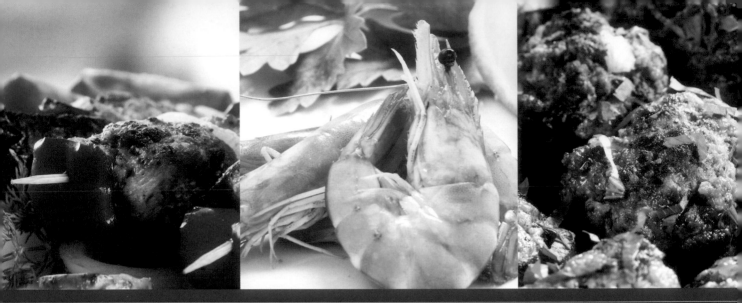

Chapter 3

Paleo Antipasti:

Small Nibbles Before a Meal

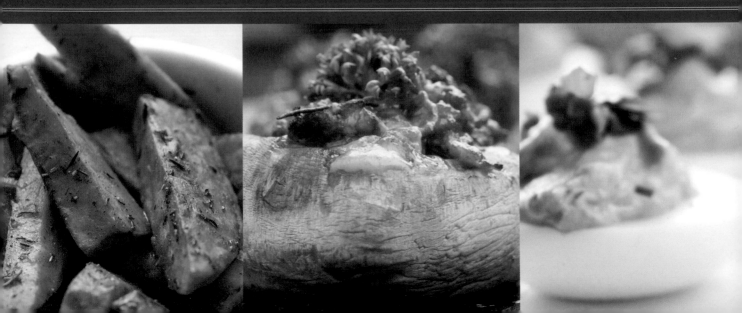

With the inherent variety and diversity of Italian cuisine, based on the influences from lands as exotic as Africa or as neighborly as France and Greece, there is no shortage of what you can put together and serve as part of your homemade antipasti, or appetizers. Italians like to combine tastes and textures, ranging from fresh vegetables to smoky pancetta-enhanced dishes. The slow cooker is your best friend when it comes to creating mini-meal marvels with Italian flare and flavor. When you make these ahead of time, you're free to focus on other entertainment preparations, like cleaning and setting the table. These recipes are simple, elegant, and healthy.

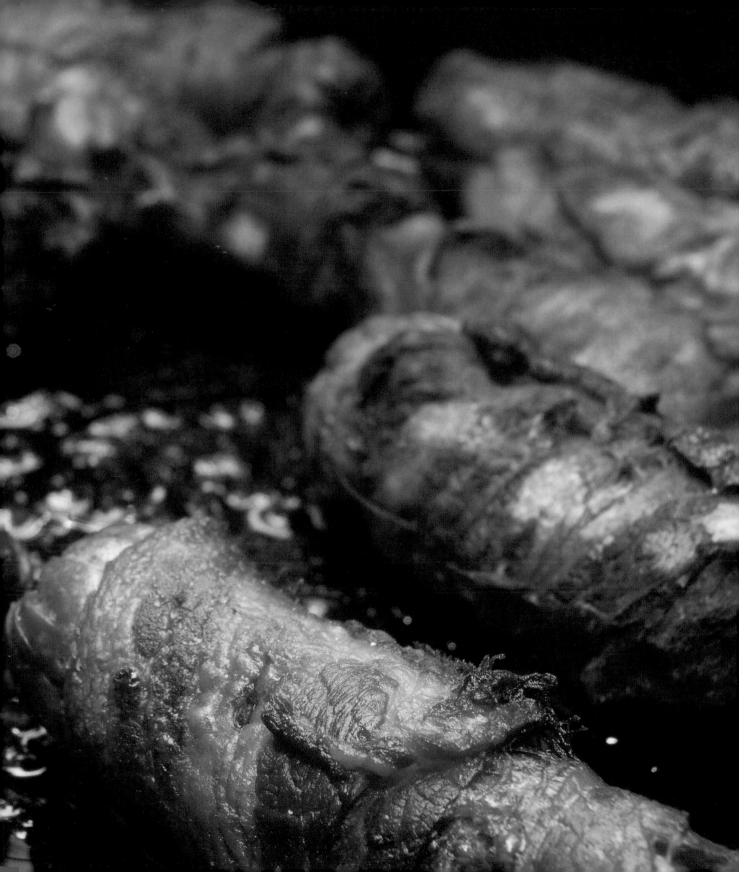

Sausage and Pancetta Wraps

These treats are a great way to indulge a craving for a fun snack. Depending on the kind of sausage you choose, the dish can take on a range of tastes.

Makes 10 to 12 party servings.

2 pounds Italian sausage
1 pound pancetta, sliced thick
Honey to drizzle

1. Work with whole sausages and individual slices of pancetta. Lay the pancetta down on a plate or piece of waxed paper, place the sausage at one end, and wrap the pancetta around the sausage, working at an angle so the pancetta covers the entire link. Secure the ends with wooden toothpicks.

2. Place the wrapped sausages in the slow cooker and drizzle lightly with honey. Stack in layers until all the sausages are in the slow cooker.

3. Cover and cook on Low for 4 to 6 hours or on High for about 2 hours. Remove with tongs, slice into bite-sized pieces, and put a toothpick into every piece to secure the pancetta and make for easy eating.

Variation:
While choosing Italian sausages is easiest—and these are available in either sweet or hot varieties—you can experiment with all different kinds of sausage. Try this recipe with seasoned chicken sausage, for example, or with pieces of kielbasa. The only kind of sausage links to avoid are those made for breakfast, as they are too small.

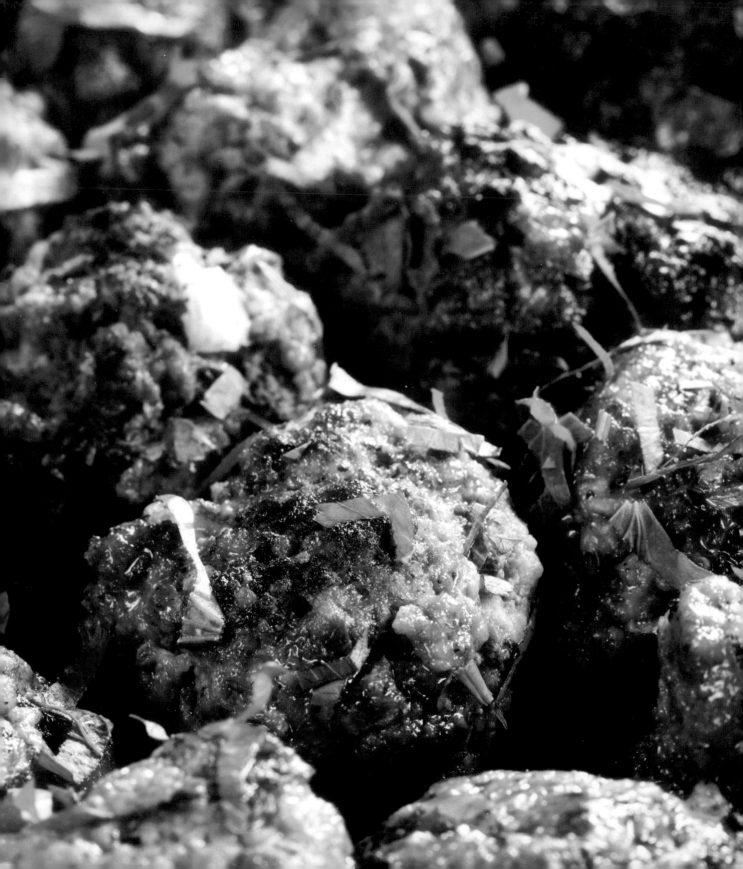

Seasoned Mini Meatballs

Always satisfying, and always a hit at parties, there's something that's just fun about meatballs. Make them for regular meals, too, to lighten up a weeknight dinner. Another great thing about them is that they freeze well!

Makes about 24 small meatballs.

2 pounds ground beef

2 teaspoons fresh thyme, chopped fine

1 teaspoon ground fennel seeds

2 tablespoons fresh parsley, minced

1 large egg, beaten

¼ onion, minced fine

2 cloves garlic, minced

1 tablespoon coconut oil

Salt and pepper to taste

1. In a large bowl, combine the ground beef, thyme, fennel seeds, parsley, egg, onion, and garlic. Stir to combine well. Form the meat mixture into meatballs and set aside on a plate.

2. In a large skillet, heat coconut oil over medium-high heat to melting. Add the meatballs (in batches if necessary) and turn them so they brown on all sides. Using a slotted spoon, transfer the browned meatballs to the slow cooker.

3. Cover and cook on Low for 3 to 4 hours, or on High for 2 to 3 hours. Sprinkle with salt and pepper before serving.

Variations:

These meatballs are delicious on their own but are sensational with dipping sauces. Try:

* A classic Italian marinara (tomato sauce).
* A barbeforte (horseradish sauce). Make a simple one by combining ½ cup ground horseradish with 2 teaspoons salt and 1½ teaspoons balsamic vinegar. While stirring these briskly (or running slowly in a food processor), add about a cup of olive oil in a drizzle.

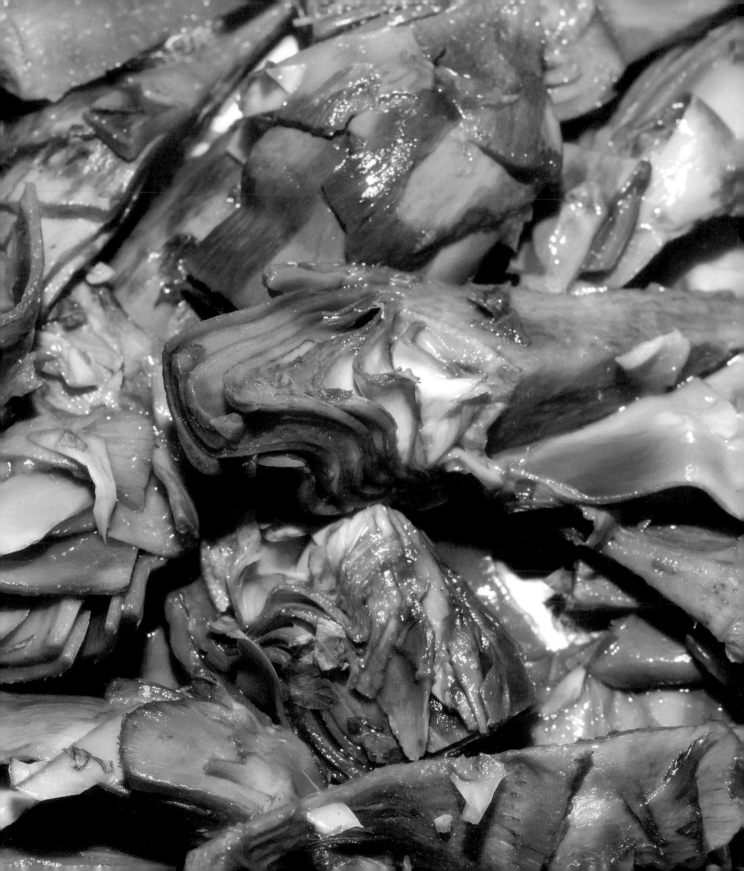

Chicken and Artichoke Wraps

A wrap is really just a way to contain the food that's inside it. While we think of wraps as being made of pastry or grains, a leaf of a fresh green makes for an equally appropriate container—and is truthfully much more flavorful.

Makes approximately two dozen appetizer wraps.

4 boneless skinless chicken breasts or thighs

2 tablespoons olive oil

3 cloves garlic, minced

¼ onion, minced

1 large carrot, coarsely chopped

1 tablespoon fresh-squeezed lemon juice

1 teaspoon lemon zest

1 tablespoon fresh parsley, minced

1 6- or 8-oz jar artichoke hearts packed in oil, drained

1 head Romaine lettuce

1. Cut the chicken into bite-sized pieces and put it in the slow cooker. In a bowl, combine the olive oil, garlic, onion, carrot, lemon juice, zest, and parsley. Pour over chicken.

2. Cover and cook on Low for 5 to 6 hours or on High for 3 to 4 hours. In the last hour of cooking, add the artichoke hearts and stir to combine. Continue cooking for the desired time, or until chicken is very tender. Stir the mix, and pull the chicken apart with a fork. Allow to cool.

3. Wash and dry 10 to 12 large Romaine leaves. Put a scoop of the shredded chicken mix onto a leaf and roll it up. Secure with a toothpick.

Variations:
There are lots of foods you can include with the chicken mixture to enhance the flavor and texture of these wraps. Try:
* Fresh anchovy filets
* Sliced almonds, toasted
* Chopped celery
* Chopped red peppers
* Green or red seedless grapes, cut in half
* Chopped parsley

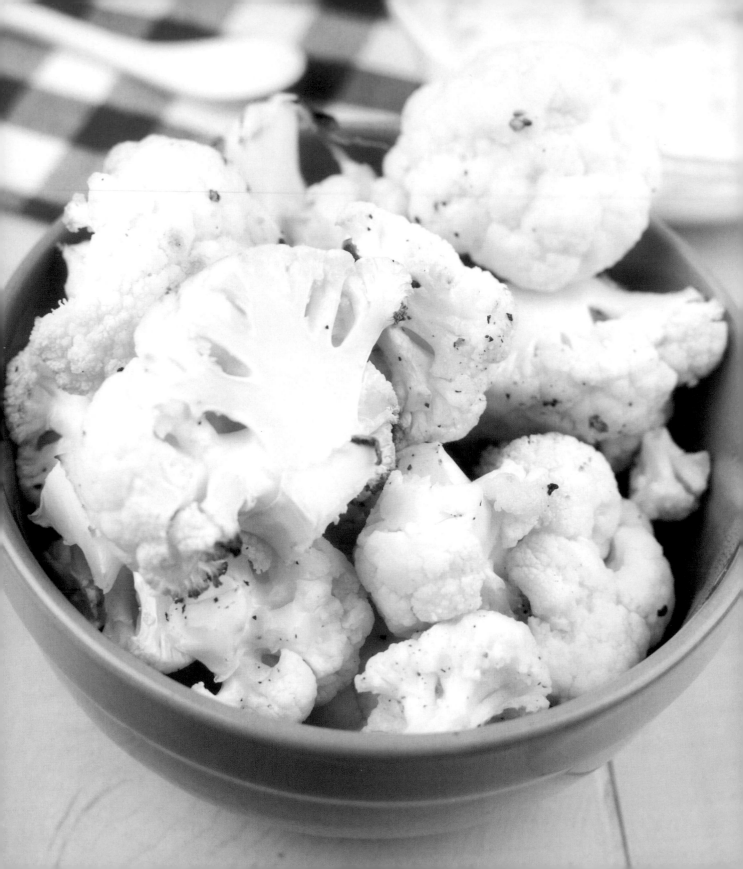

Cauliflower Italiano

Really easy to make, and really tasty! Vary the amounts of the spices if you lean more toward the flavor of one over another.

Makes about 3 cups.

1 head cauliflower
Olive oil for drizzling
Freshly ground pepper
Sea salt
1 clove minced garlic
Minced fresh oregano
Minced fresh parsley

1. Core the cauliflower and break the head up into florets. You can trim and cut the stems into bite-sized pieces, as well.

2. Put the pieces into the slow cooker. Drizzle with olive oil so that there is a light coating of oil on the cauliflower. Season the oiled cauliflower with the pepper and salt, add the garlic, and stir.

3. Cover and cook on Low for 4 hours, or on High for 2 hours. Sprinkle the cauliflower with the fresh herbs, just so the florets and stems are covered. Put the cover back on and continue to cook for another 30 to 60 minutes until the cauliflower is tender. Serve in a bowl with long toothpicks.

Variation:
For a more colorful dish, replace half of the head of cauliflower with half a head of broccoli.

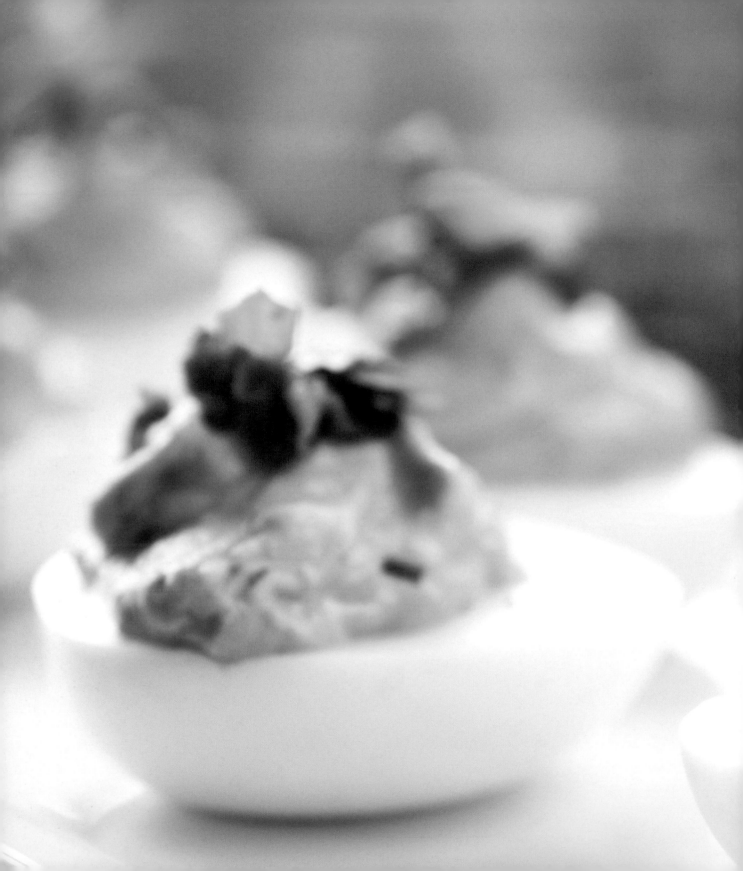

Herbed Eggs

The flavors in the yolk mixture of this Italian take on deviled eggs is so good that these may become your new go-to recipe for this simple appetizer. Slow-cooking eggs is as simple as it gets, and unlike hard-boiling your eggs on the stovetop, you don't have to worry about the water boiling over.

Makes 16 to 24 egg halves.

8 to 12 eggs (depending on how many fit in one layer on the bottom of your slow cooker)

Large bowl of ice water

2 tablespoons chopped fresh parsley

4 capers, minced

4 anchovy filets

2 cloves garlic, pressed through a garlic press

¼ cup olive oil

Salt and pepper to taste

Bits of bacon for garnish, if desired

1. Place the eggs gently on the bottom of the slow cooker, being sure they are in a single layer. Add tap water to cover. Cover and cook on High for 2 hours.

2. When cooked, remove with tongs and place into bowl of ice water. Let the eggs stay in the ice bath for a couple of minutes. This reduces the temperature and loosens the shell for easy peeling.

3. Once peeled, cut the eggs in half and scoop out the cooked yolks into a large bowl. Mash them with a fork so they are crumbled but not too finely mashed.

4. In a smaller bowl or in a small food processor, combine the parsley, capers, anchovy filets, and garlic. Mash with a fork or combine on low with the food processor, drizzling in the oil to form a creamy paste. Add the paste to the egg yolks and stir to combine. Season with salt and pepper. Fill the cooked whites with the mixture. Garnish with bacon if desired. Refrigerate until ready to serve.

> Fresh anchovy filets taste much different from the over-salted anchovies most Americans are used to. You can buy them at specialty shops or from a fresh fish market. If you really don't like anchovies, just leave them out of the mix. You may need to add a bit more olive oil.

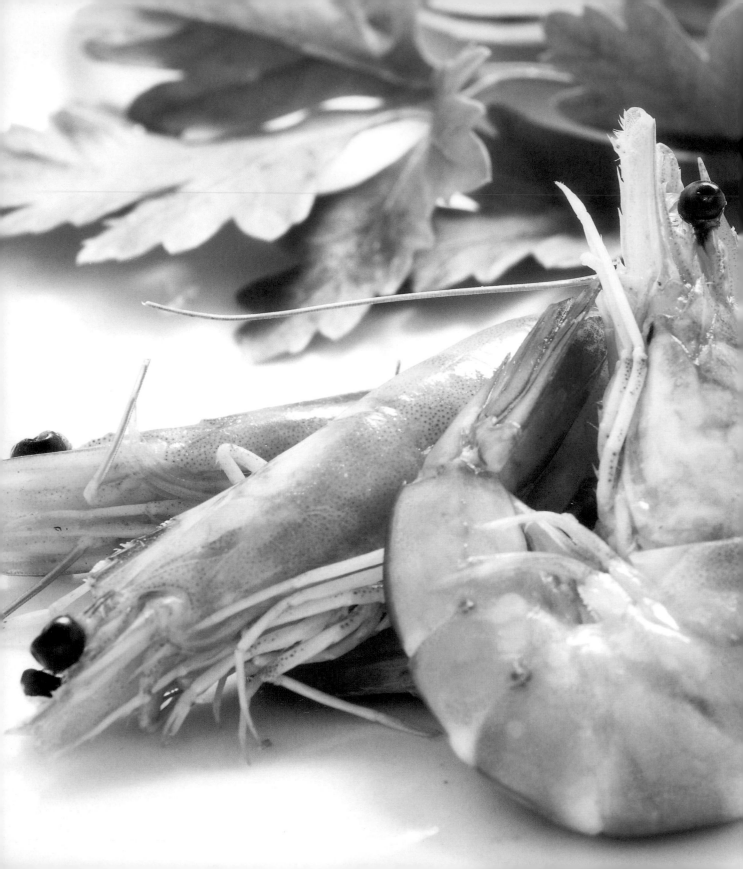

Simple and Elegant Gambretti (Shrimp)

Use the slow cooker to poach the shrimp, and then stir the warm seafood in the oil and lemon mixture. Close your eyes and imagine yourself on the Adriatic coast of Italy. You've arrived!

Makes 4 to 8 appetizers.

12 cups water

¼ bulb fennel, leaves removed and cut into thick strips

1 small carrot, peeled

1 tablespoon white wine vinegar

½ cup freshly squeezed lemon juice (seeds removed). It's important to use the juice of freshly squeezed lemons for the best flavor.

½ cup extra virgin olive oil (the fruitier the better)

2 pounds small fresh shrimp, uncooked, shells on

1 teaspoon fresh parsley, minced

Sea salt and freshly ground pepper to taste

1. Put the water, fennel, carrot, and vinegar in the slow cooker. If you plan to serve the shrimp sooner rather than later, turn the cooker on High and let the vegetables poach for about 3 hours. If you want to do this while you're out for the day, put the cooker on Low and leave it for 6 to 8 hours. The water should be very hot—if it was on the stove, it would be close to boiling.

2. While the vegetables are poaching, prepare the lemon and oil mixture by combining them in a medium-sized bowl and stirring with a whisk. Set the mixture aside.

3. When the water in the slow cooker is very hot, remove the poached vegetables and add the shrimp.

4. Cover and cook on High for 10 to 30 minutes. Check after 10 minutes, and every 5 minutes thereafter. Cooking time will depend on the size of the shrimp. When cooked, the shrimp will turn pink and firm but not hard. It's important not to overcook them.

5. When cooked, drain the shrimp and peel them, placing the warm, peeled shrimp in the bowl with the oil and lemon mixture. When all the shrimp have been added, stir, sprinkle with parsley, season with salt and pepper, and serve immediately.

A slow cooker is not meant to boil things—water, gravy, stew, anything! That's one of the great things about it and is why you don't have to worry about leaving it on all day. When it comes to a recipe like this, where you want to cook something quickly in a hot liquid, you need to factor in the time it's going to take for the broth to get very hot. Another benefit to this method is that you have more flexibility with the cooking time of the shrimp and don't have to worry as much about them rapidly overcooking.

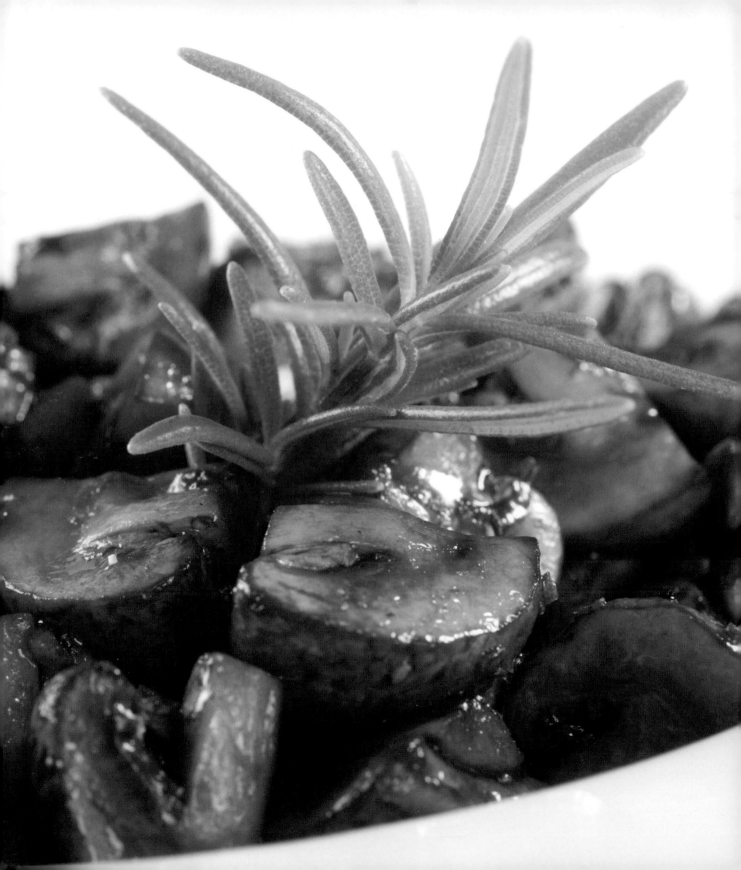

Baby Bellos with Rosemary

There's nothing like a big slice of slow-cooked Portobello mushroom, when the flavor explodes with every bite. This is another so simple but so satisfying recipe that can easily be doubled to make extra. You'll want to be able to quickly reheat them to enjoy through the week.

Makes about 2 cups cooked Portobellos.

2 lbs baby Portobellos or a similar quantity of large Portobellos cut into chunks

3 tablespoons olive oil

3 tablespoons ghee or clarified butter

Salt and pepper to taste

1 teaspoon chopped fresh rosemary

1. Go over the Portobellos and remove any obvious dirt by brushing or shaking it off. Slice the tough stems off, and cut the mushrooms in half. Put the pieces into the slow cooker.

2. In a small skillet, heat the olive oil and ghee over medium heat until melted and combined. Pour the melted oil/butter combo over the Portobellos.

3. Cover and cook on Low for 3 to 4 hours or on High for 1 to 2 hours. The mushrooms should be cooked through but not too mushy. Season lightly with salt and pepper before serving, and sprinkle with fresh rosemary.

The Portobello mushroom is an oversized crimini mushroom. Both are dark brown mushrooms related to the common mushroom. Creminis and Portobellos share a mustier, earthier flavor as well as color from the common white mushroom. Large Portobellos are so meaty that they are often cooked as meat substitutes, making great "burgers" for vegetarians.

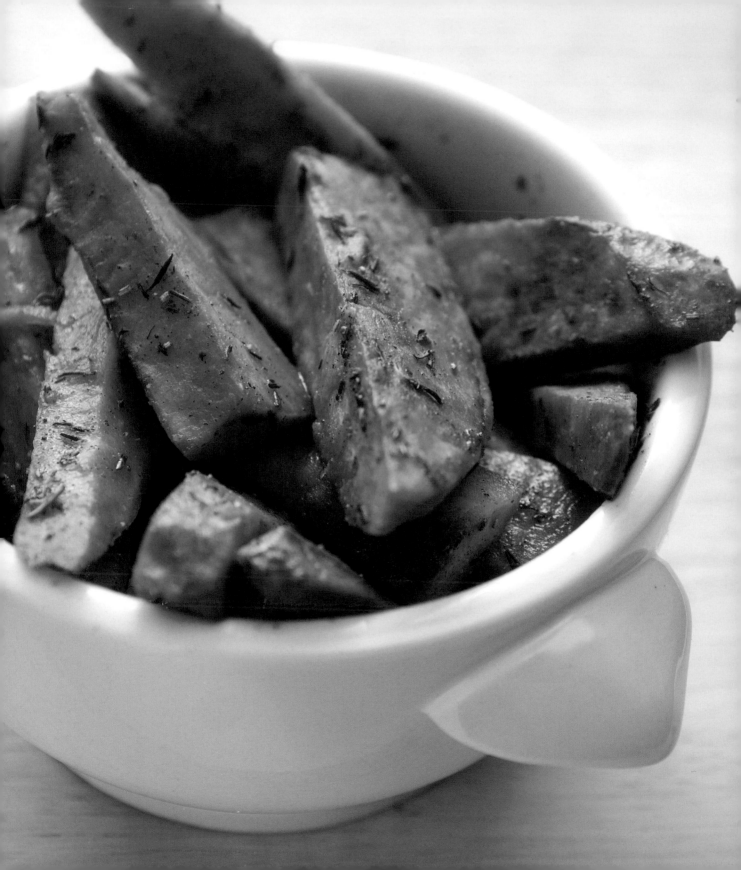

Sweet Potato Wedges

This vegetable—rich in Vitamin A, beta-carotene, and an assortment of minerals—has been rapidly replacing the white potato in lots of recipes, including French fries, which is the basis of this snack. Going Italian with the seasoning adds even more vitamins.

Makes 4 to 6 servings.

4 medium-sized sweet potatoes, peeled and sliced into thin wedges

½ cup water

4 tablespoons coconut oil

Salt and pepper

1 tablespoon fresh parsley, chopped

2 or 3 leaves of fresh basil, chopped

1. Place the sweet potato wedges into the slow cooker. Add the water. Drizzle the sweet potatoes with the oil. Cover and cook on Low for 4 to 5 hours or on High for 2 to 3 hours.

2. Prop open the lid with the handle of a wooden spoon, and continue to cook another 30 minutes or so on High to get some browning.

3. When ready to serve, season with salt and pepper, then top with the chopped fresh herbs.

Variation:

One thing you may really develop a liking for while working with the recipes in this cookbook is fresh anchovies. If you become addicted, you can add some zing to this dish, too, by mashing a couple of fresh anchovy filets into the olive oil used to drizzle the sweet potatoes.

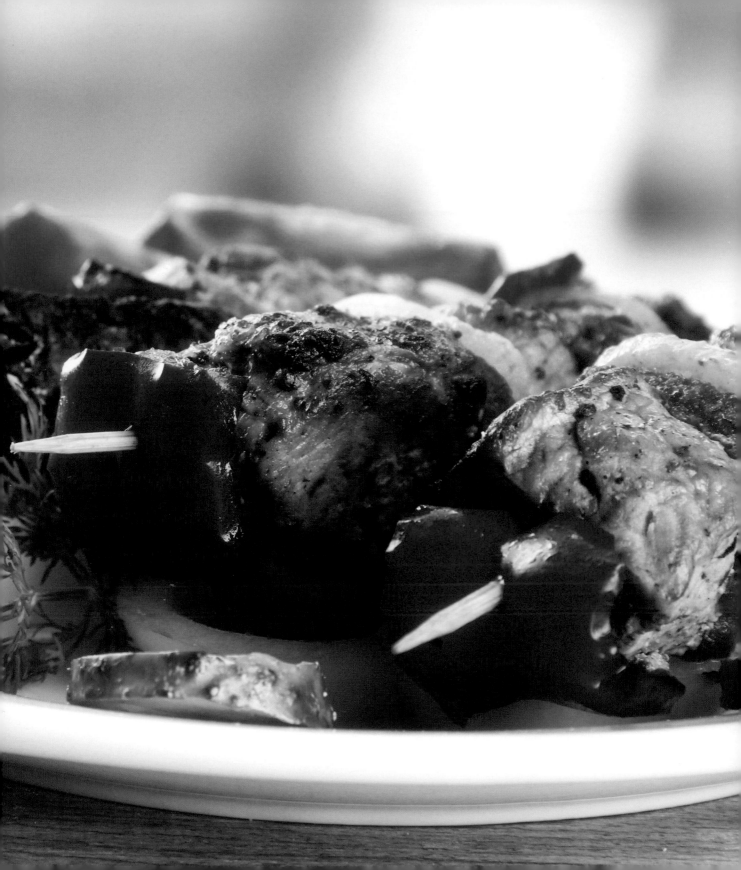

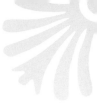

Lamb Kabobs

You'll be eager to eat these when you smell them cooking. This is a recipe full of Southern Mediterranean goodness.

Makes 6 to 10 kabobs.

½ cup olive oil

1 teaspoon rosemary, minced

3 cloves garlic, minced

¼ teaspoon each salt and pepper

1 pound boneless leg of lamb, cubed

2 red bell peppers, cored and seeded, cut into chunks

1 onion, peeled and cut into small wedges

1 large zucchini, cut into thick slices

Wooden skewer sticks, broken to fit the length of the slow cooker

1. In a large bowl, combine the olive oil, rosemary, garlic, and salt and pepper. Add the lamb cubes and stir to coat.

2. Using the wooden skewers, make kabobs alternating lamb, peppers, onions, and zucchini.

3. Lay the kabobs in the slow cooker, and pour the remaining oil mixture over them.

4. Cover and cook on Low for 3 to 4 hours or on High for 1 to 2 hours until lamb is cooked through and vegetables have softened. Baste with juices from the slow cooker before serving.

Lamb is eaten much more around the world than in the United States, where beef is king. It is in central Italy where you can find hilltops dotted with flocks of lambs and their shepherds—and where cooking with lamb is a family tradition.

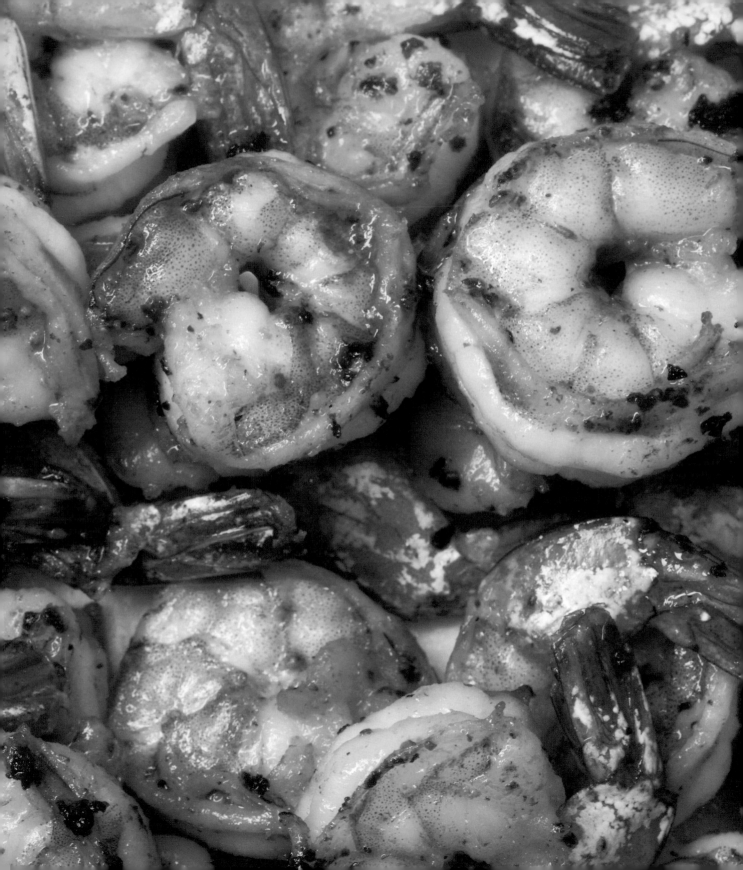

Spicy Shrimp Scampi

This is a flavorful primi that is incredibly easy to make and always a hit. It's redolent with garlic, spicy from crushed red pepper, and brightly colored from a combination of paprika and parsley.

Makes 4 to 6 servings.

½ cup olive oil

6 garlic cloves, minced

1 tablespoon paprika

2 pounds extra-large shrimp (16-20/pound), peeled and deveined

½ cup dry white wine

3 tablespoons fresh parsley, chopped

Salt and crushed red pepper flakes to taste

Lemon wedges for serving

1. Combine olive oil, garlic, paprika, shrimp, wine, and parsley in the slow cooker.

2. Cook on Low for 3 to 4 hours or on High for 1½ to 2 hours, or until shrimp are pink and cooked through. Season to taste with salt and red pepper flakes.

3. Serve warm or at room temperature, and pass lemon wedges separately.

Note: The dish can be prepared up to 1 day in advance and refrigerated, tightly covered with plastic wrap. Allow it to sit at room temperature for 30 minutes before serving.

When you buy shrimp that are still in their shells, they need to be peeled, and that's an obvious task. Step two is to devein them. In one hand, hold the shrimp with its back facing up. With the other hand, cut gently down the back with a small paring knife. If there is a thin black line, scrape it out. That's the "vein"—it's actually the intestinal tract—which can be bitter and gritty.

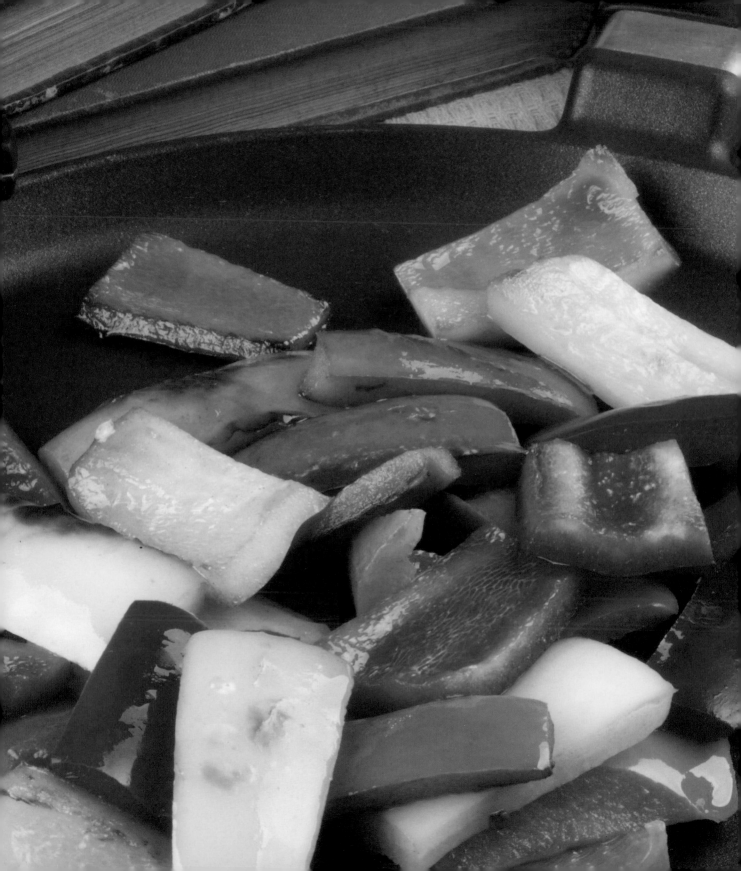

Peperonata (Roasted Peppers)

Roasted peppers are succulent and delicious. Slow cooking with some tomatoes, herbs, and a hint of balsamic vinegar renders the vegetables nearly sweet. These are delicious as a snack or as a topping for cooked meat or fish.

Makes 1½ cups.

⅓ cup olive oil

2 large onions, halved and thinly sliced

1 large green bell pepper, seeds and ribs removed, and thinly sliced

1 large red bell pepper, seeds and ribs removed, and thinly sliced

1 large orange or yellow bell pepper, seeds and ribs removed, and thinly sliced

2 garlic cloves, minced

2 ripe plum tomatoes, cored, seeded, and diced

3 tablespoons chicken broth or stock

2 tablespoons fresh rosemary, chopped

2 tablespoons balsamic vinegar

Salt and pepper to taste

1. Heat oil in a large skillet over medium-high heat. Add onions, all the sliced peppers, and the garlic. Cook, stirring frequently, for 3 minutes, or until onions are translucent. Scrape mixture into the slow cooker.

2. Add tomatoes, stock, and rosemary to the slow cooker, and stir well. Cook on Low for 4 to 5 hours or on High for 2 to 2½ hours, or until peppers are very tender.

3. Stir in vinegar, and season to taste with salt and pepper.

> It's easier to slice and dice bell peppers from the inside out. Once the seeds and ribs have been removed, place the shiny, slippery skin on your cutting board, and you'll find it's easier to control your knife and cut the size pieces you desire.

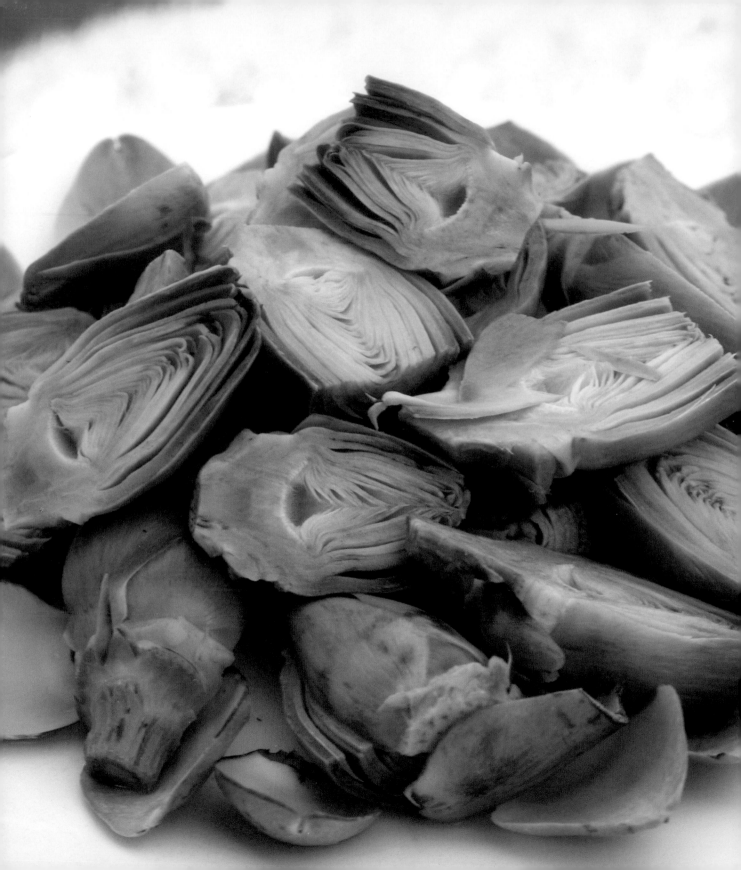

Braised Baby Artichokes with Prosciutto

Thankfully, it's now fairly easy to find baby artichokes in North American supermarkets. With the baby artichokes, the entire vegetable is edible, so you don't have to remove the hairy "choke." This makes preparation much simpler.

Makes 8 to 10 servings.

2 lemons

24 baby artichokes

3 tablespoons olive oil

3 shallots, diced

2 cloves garlic, minced

½ cup prosciutto, chopped

¼ cup chicken stock or broth

½ cup dry white wine

2 tablespoons freshly squeezed lemon juice (seeds removed)

½ teaspoon dried thyme

1 bay leaf

2 tablespoons ghee

Salt and pepper to taste

Fresh chopped parsley for garnish

1. Place 6 cups of very cold tap water in a large mixing bowl, squeeze in juice from lemons, and add lemon halves.

2. Work on 1 artichoke at a time because they discolor very quickly. If there is a stem, trim and peel the dark green skin from the stem. Break off all the small, dark leaves on the bottom so that the artichoke resembles a rose bud. Cut off the top 1 inch, and then cut them in half lengthwise. Place in the lemon water, and repeat until all artichokes are trimmed.

3. Heat oil in a large skillet over medium-high heat. Add shallots, garlic, and prosciutto, and cook, stirring frequently, for 3 minutes, or until shallots are translucent. Drain artichokes and add them to the skillet along with stock, wine, lemon juice, thyme, and bay leaf. Bring to a boil, and transfer mixture to the slow cooker.

4. Cook on Low for 3 to 4 hours or on High for 1½ to 2 hours, or until artichokes are very tender. Add ghee to the slow cooker, and cook until melted.

5. Remove and discard bay leaf. Season with salt and pepper to taste. Sprinkle with fresh parsley when serving.

Variation:
Toasted pine nuts are an excellent complement to this dish, as they add a buttery crunchiness to it, and the flavors pair perfectly. To toast the pine nuts, put them in a heavy clad or non-stick skillet and heat them over medium heat. Stir with a wooden spoon while they heat, taking care not to overdo them. The process takes 3 to 5 minutes.

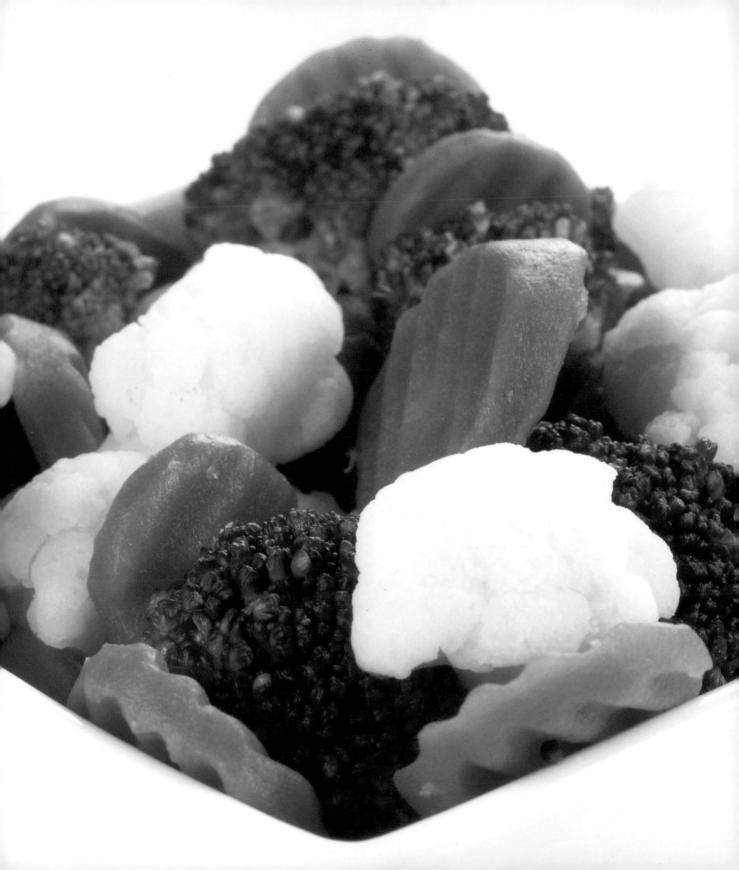

Steamed and Seasoned Vegetables

These are a typical addition to an antipasti platter. They're easy to make and full of fresh, seasonal goodness.

Makes 8 to 10 servings.

2 carrots, thickly sliced

½ head cauliflower, broken into florets

1 broccoli crown, broken into florets

¼ pound mixed brine-cured olives

¼ cup freshly squeezed lemon juice (seeds removed)

1 teaspoon dried oregano

¼ teaspoon crushed red pepper flakes

Salt to taste

½ cup olive oil

1. Place a steamer basket in the slow cooker, and layer the vegetables with the carrots on the bottom, then the cauliflower, then the broccoli. Add ½ cup water to the slow cooker, and cook vegetables on Low for 3 to 5 hours or on High for 1½ to 2 hours, or until they are crisp-tender.

2. Fill a large bowl with cold tap water and some ice cubes. When the vegetables are ready, lift the steamer basket and place it into the bowl of ice water. This will stop the cooking and set the color. Drain the vegetables in a colander, and put them in a mixing bowl with the olives.

3. Combine the lemon juice, oregano, red pepper flakes, and salt in a jar with a tight-fitting lid, and shake well. Add olive oil, and shake well again.

4. Pour over the vegetables and toss to coat. Allow to rest for about 15 minutes before serving, tossing them a few more times to distribute the dressing. Serve at room temperature.

> Steaming preserves more of the vegetables' natural nutrients than boiling. The vitamins and minerals are leached into the hot water when they're boiled.

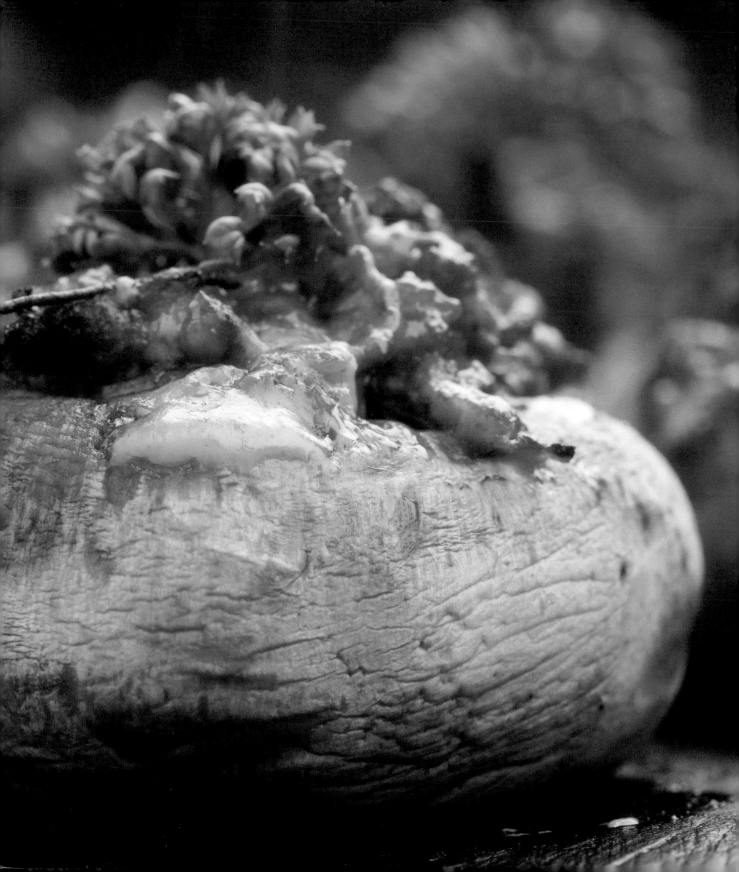

Stuffed Mushrooms

These are so tasty! Filled with lots of herbs and some smoky pancetta, they are the first appetizers to disappear from the table.

Makes 4 to 6 servings.

1 pound large white mushrooms

½ cup chopped Portobello mushroom

¼ pound pancetta or thick-cut bacon, chopped fine

4 fresh anchovy filets, minced

2 cloves garlic, pressed

1 egg

3 tablespoons fresh parsley, chopped

¼ cup almond meal

¼ cup golden flax meal

1 teaspoon arrowroot

Olive oil for drizzling

1. Clean the large white mushrooms to be stuffed by dabbing at them to remove any dirt with a wet paper towel. If the mushrooms have stems, remove them gently. When cleaned, place them cap side down in the slow cooker.

2. In a large mixing bowl, combine the chopped Portobello mushroom, pancetta, anchovies, garlic, egg, and parsley. Stir with a fork to combine, further mashing it into a somewhat fine-textured mix. Season with salt and pepper. Stuff the mushroom caps with the mixture.

3. In a small bowl, combine the almond and flax meals and the arrowroot. Sprinkle this liberally over the stuffed mushrooms. Drizzle with some olive oil.

4. Cook on Low for 4 to 6 Hours or on High for 2 to 3 hours until the mushrooms are tender and the filling is cooked. Remove the stuffed mushrooms carefully and serve on a platter. Garnish with additional fresh parsley if desired. Reserve the liquid to add to soup.

Stuffed mushrooms typically contain bread crumbs, which help hold the stuffing together. The combination of almond and golden flax meals, with some arrowroot added to help thicken the grain mix, is a wonderful Paleo substitute—and healthy, to boot!

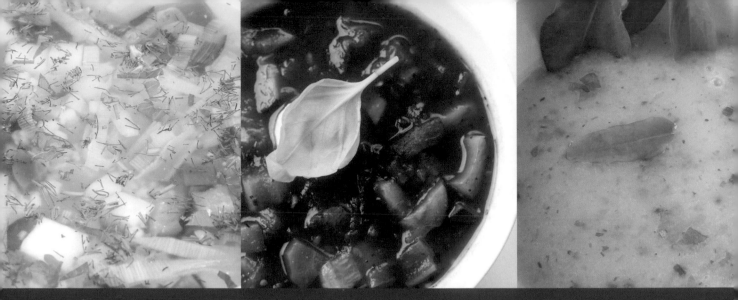

Chapter 4

Paleo Minestre:

Soups and Sauces

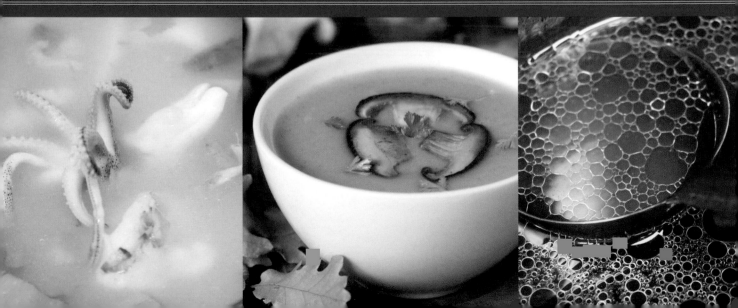

*A*ll cuisines savor homemade soups, and it's easy to understand why! They're typically easy to make, include foods that tend to be plentiful, can be readily tweaked to accentuate a particular flavor or ingredient, and best of all, they taste great and are so good for you. Italian cuisine is no exception, and this collection of soups—and sauces—demonstrates the freshness and inherent goodness that make them all *delicioso!* Being a fan of artichokes from the time I was little, I especially love that this vegetable is prevalent in Italian cooking, including soups and sauces.

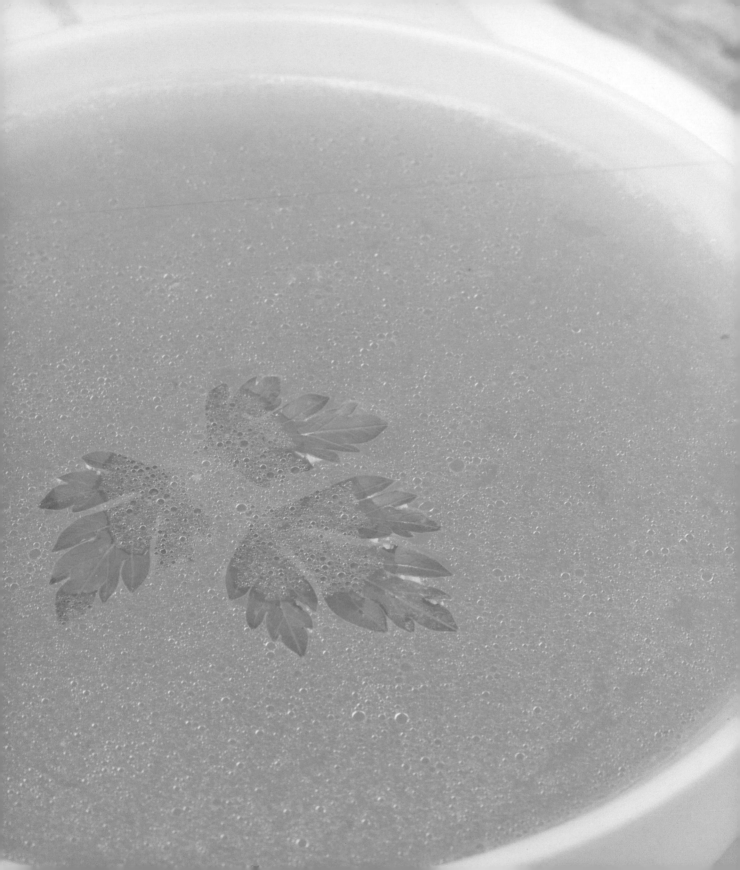

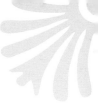

Chicken Stock

Besides being the base of so many recipes, homemade stock is in and of itself an amazing food. Made with all parts of the chicken (or beef, or fish), a slow-cooked stock is rich in many minerals essential to good health, including calcium, magnesium, phosphorous, silicon, sulphur, and even glucosamine and chondroitin, which we often pay a lot of money for as a supplement for joint care! It is prized around the world as a remedy for whatever ails you, from digestive upset to sore throats to low libido. (Note: The amounts in this recipe are for a larger slow cooker; if yours is small, cut the recipe in half.)

Stock can be stored in the refrigerator for several days, or kept frozen.

1 whole free-range chicken,
or 2 to 3 pounds of the bony parts
(necks, backs, breastbones, legs, wings)

Gizzards from the chicken

2 to 4 chicken feet (optional but beneficial)

4 quarts cold water

2 tablespoons vinegar

1 large onion, chopped

2 carrots, peeled and sliced

2 celery stalks, chopped

1 bunch parsley, chopped

1. If you are using a whole chicken, cut off the neck, wings, and legs and cut them into pieces. Cut the rest of the chicken pieces into chunks.

2. Place chicken pieces in the slow cooker and top with all vegetables except the parsley. Cover with water and vinegar. Cover, and let the meat and vegetables sit in the liquid for 30 minutes to 1 hour.

3. Turn the slow cooker to High and cook for 2 to 3 hours, or until boiling. Remove the cover and spoon off and discard any "scum" that has risen to the top.

4. Replace the cover and reduce the heat to Low. Cook for 8 to 10 hours. Add the parsley in the last 15 minutes or so.

5. When cooking is complete, remove the solids with a slotted spoon into a colander over a bowl. Any drippings in the bowl can go back into the stock. Remove any meat from the bones and eat separately. Transfer the stock to a large bowl and refrigerate. When the fat is congealed on top, remove it, and transfer the stock to several smaller containers with tight-fitting lids.

Variation:

For a browner, even richer stock, place the chicken pieces on a cookie sheet. Preheat the oven broiler, and broil for about 3 minutes per side, until browned.

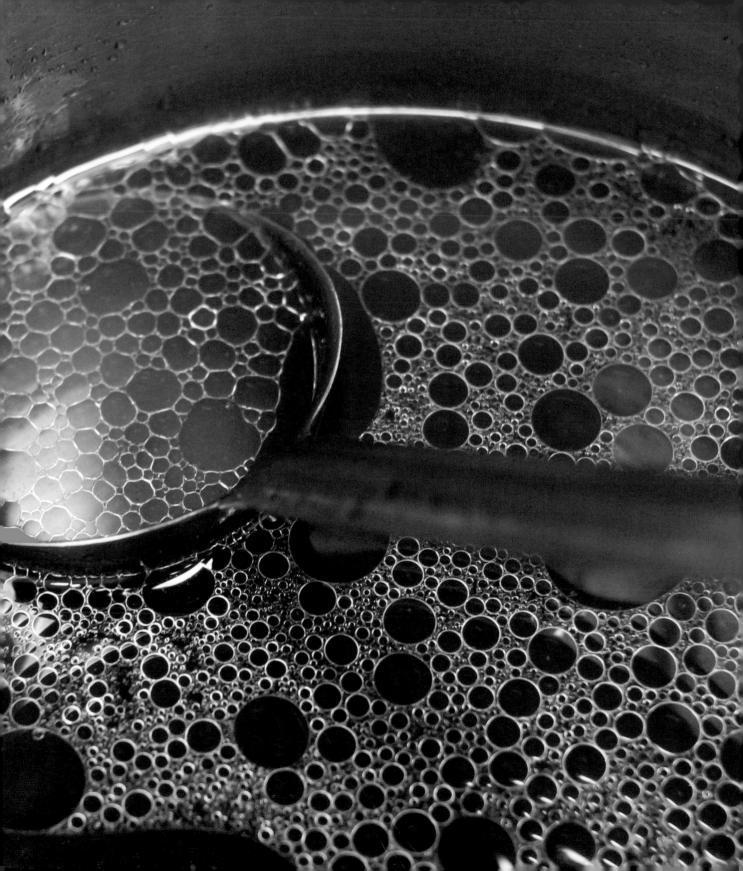

Beef Stock

This stock will add new layers of delicious complexity to the recipes it's in—and will make your kitchen smell fantastic while it's cooking.

Stock can be stored in the refrigerator for several days, or kept frozen.

2 pounds beef marrow bones

3 quarts water

¼ cup vinegar

2 pounds meaty rib or neck bones

1 large onion, chopped

2 large carrots, chopped

2 celery stalks, chopped

3 sprigs of fresh thyme

1 teaspoon peppercorns

1 bunch parsley

1. Place the beef bones in a large pot and cover with water and vinegar. Let stand for one hour.

2. Place the meaty bones in a roasting pan. Preheat the oven to 350 and roast until well browned, about 30 to 40 minutes.

3. Place the soaked beef bones and the browned pieces in the slow cooker. Add the vegetables, thyme, and peppercorns, and cover with the water.

4. Discard the fat from the roasting pan, and fill with an inch or so of water. Place the pan over a burner on medium-high heat, and as the water heats, stir to loosen the coagulated juices and browned bits. Add this to the slow cooker. The water should just cover the meat and vegetables; add more if it doesn't.

5. Turn the slow cooker on High and cook for 2 to 3 hours until liquid is boiling. Remove lid and scoop out and discard scum that has risen to the top.

6. Replace the lid, lower the heat to Low, and cook for 12 to 18 hours—the longer, the better. Add the parsley during the last 15 minutes.

7. When cooking is complete, remove the solids with a slotted spoon into a colander over a bowl. Any drippings in the bowl can go back into the stock. Remove any meat from the bones and eat separately. Transfer the stock to a large bowl and refrigerate. When the fat is congealed on top, remove it, and transfer the stock to several smaller containers with tight-fitting lids.

Making broths is Paleo at its purest. After all, nothing was wasted from a slaughtered animal in Paleolithic times—and even still in many parts of the world. The nutrients extracted from the slow-cooking process are easily absorbed by the body. It's wonderful to get so much goodness out of parts we might normally discard.

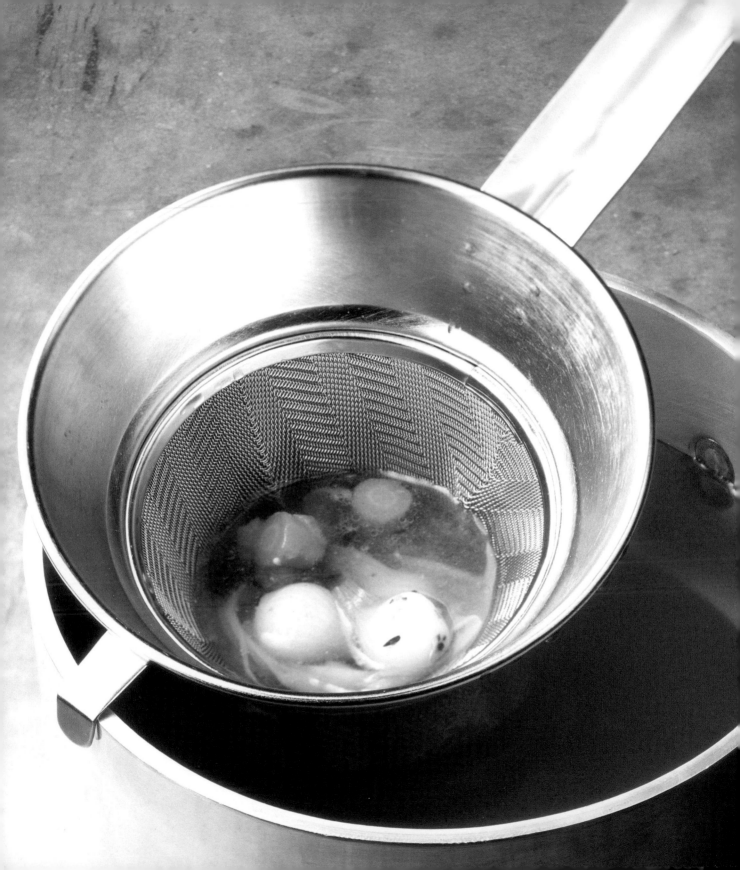

Vegetable Stock

Even if you're cooking a vegetarian dish, it's important to start with the vegetable stock rather than adding more vegetables to the dish. It creates the background for all other flavors.

Stock can be stored in the refrigerator for several days, or kept frozen.

2 quarts boiling water

2 carrots, thinly sliced

2 stalks celery, chopped

2 large leeks, white parts only, thinly sliced

1 small onion, thinly sliced

1 tablespoon black peppercorns

2 cloves garlic, peeled

3 sprigs thyme

1 bay leaf

1 bunch parsley

1. Pour boiling water into the slow cooker, and add carrots, celery, leeks, onion, peppercorns, garlic, thyme, and bay leaf. Cook on low for 6 to 8 hours or on High for 4 to 5 hours. Add parsley to final 15 minutes of cooking time.

2. Strain stock through a sieve into a large mixing bowl. Press down on the solids with the back of a spoon to extract as much liquid as possible. Discard solids.

3. Refrigerate the stock. When the fat is congealed on top, remove it, and transfer the stock to several smaller containers with tight-fitting lids.

> Save the water you use when boiling or steaming mildly flavored vegetables such as spinach, carrots or green beans, and make them part of the liquid used for the stock. However, the water from any member of the cabbage family, like broccoli or cauliflower, is too strong.

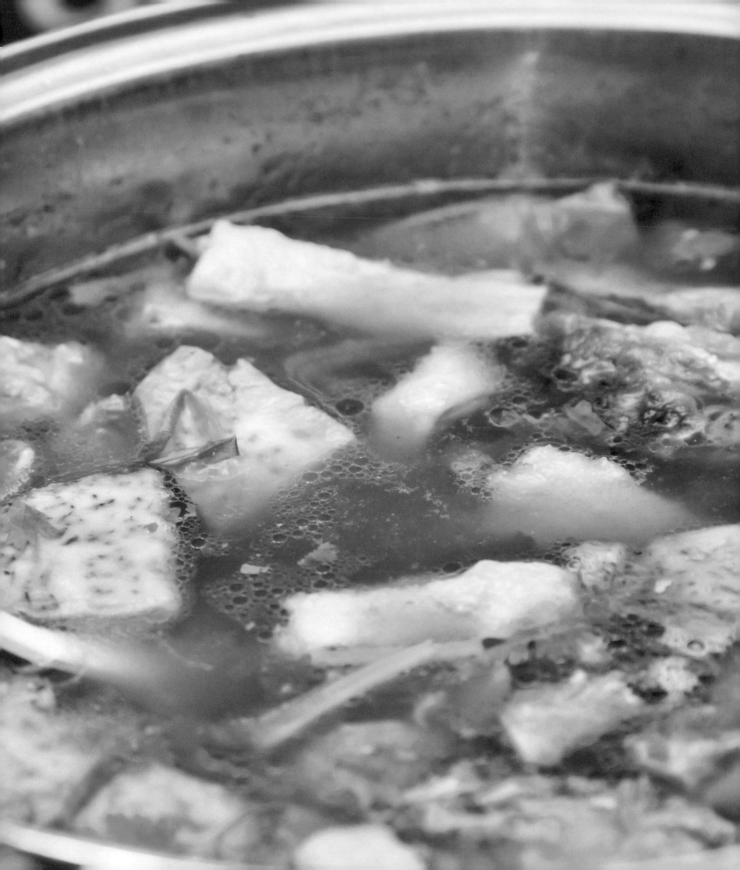

Fish Stock

The carcasses of fish typically have the filets removed already. If you can find a good fishmonger near you, you should be able to buy fish carcasses at a modest price. Be sure to get the heads, too, as they are rich in iodine and fat-soluble vitamins.

Stock can be stored in the refrigerator for several days, or kept frozen.

2 tablespoons clarified butter

2 onions, chopped

1 carrot, chopped

3 sprigs fresh thyme

Several sprigs fresh parsley

1 bay leaf

½ cup dry vermouth

2 or 3 whole carcasses from non-oily fish such as snapper, rockfish, sole or cod

¼ cup vinegar

3 quarts cold water

1. In a large skillet over medium heat, melt butter and add onions and carrots. Cook for a couple of minutes at the higher heat to coat the vegetables, then reduce the heat to low and cook, stirring occasionally, until vegetables are soft, about 30 minutes. Add the vermouth and increase the heat to bring to a near boil.

2. Place the carcasses in the slow cooker. Cover with the water and vinegar. Add the vegetable mixture. Cover and cook on High for 4 to 5 hours until liquid is boiling.

3. Remove the cover and scoop off and discard the scum that has risen to the top. Replace the cover and cook on Low for 10 to 18 hours—the longer the better.

4. When cooking is complete, remove the solids with a slotted spoon. Transfer the stock to a large bowl and refrigerate. When the fat is congealed on top, remove it, and transfer the stock to several smaller containers with tight-fitting lids.

To make Seafood Stock: Make a more delicate seafood stock using lobster bodies from which the claws and tail have been removed. For this recipe, use 3 to 4 lobster bodies, or the bodies of 2 lobsters and the shells from 2 to 4 pounds of raw shrimp.

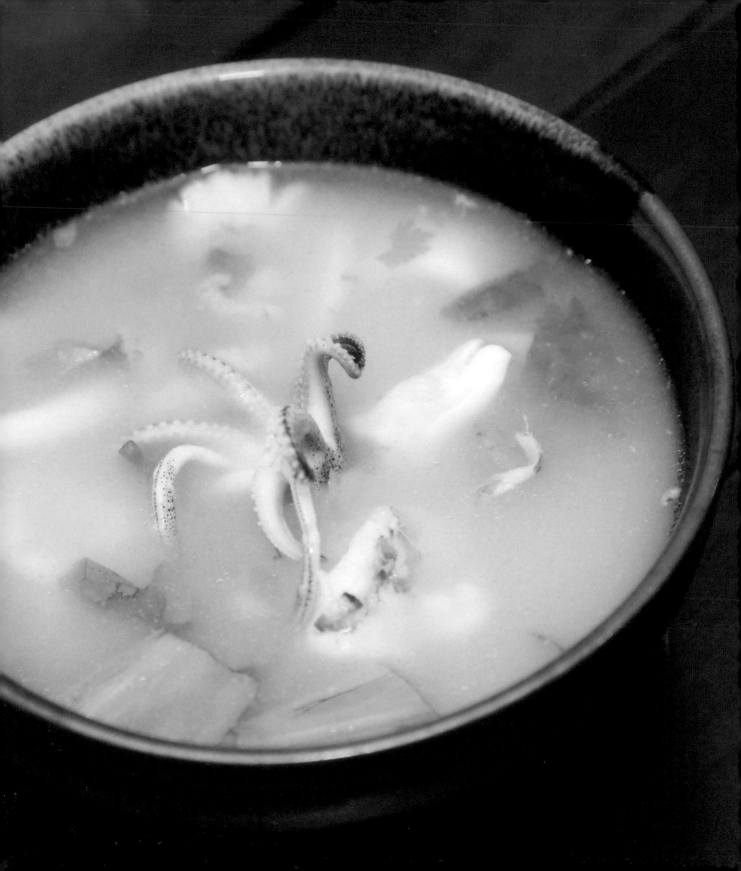

Artichoke Soup with Squid

This is an inspiration from Marcella Hazan's cookbook *Essentials of Classic Italian Cooking*. I love how Hazan identifies certain ingredients and flavors that are synonymous with Italian cooking, but says in essence it's what happens in a region—or in a family—that makes a dish special.

Makes 4 to 6 servings.

1 pound fresh or frozen whole squid (thawed if frozen)

½ cup olive oil

2 cloves garlic, minced

3 tablespoons fresh parsley, minced

1 cup dry white wine

2 medium-sized artichokes

Juice from ½ lemon

Salt and pepper to taste

1. Rinse the squid in cold water and cut into ½-inch slices. Pat dry with paper towels.

2. In a large saucepan, heat the olive oil and garlic over medium heat, stirring, until the garlic is translucent, about 3 minutes. Stir in the parsley, and add the squid, stirring to coat well with the garlic, oil, and herbs.

3. Transfer the mixture to the slow cooker. Pour the wine over the squid. Add water to cover the mixture by about 1 to 2 inches. Cook on Low for 5 to 6 hours or on High for 3 to 4 hours, until squid is tender.

4. While the squid is cooking, prepare the artichokes. Cut the stem to about ½ inch in length. Peel away the tough bottom leaves, and, working up the artichoke, continue to cut away the top parts of the leaves. When you are about halfway up, you'll have a cone of inner leaves. Cut this cone off, and carefully remove the prickly inner leaves and the fuzzy "choke" inside the artichoke, being careful not to scoop away the flesh below the fuzz. Slice the remaining artichoke into thin slices. Place the slices in a bowl of cold water to cover, and squeeze the lemon over them.

5. When the squid is tender, drain and rinse the artichoke slices. Before adding them to the squid, season the squid with salt, stirring. Add the artichoke slices. Add enough water to cover everything by about 2 inches, and then stir thoroughly. Cover and cook on Low for an additional 4 hours or on High for another 1 to 2 hours, until the artichokes are tender. Season with additional salt, if desired, and freshly ground pepper and parsley.

This is an elegant soup to serve for a dinner party, and is quite filling. It pairs beautifully with a salad as a main course.

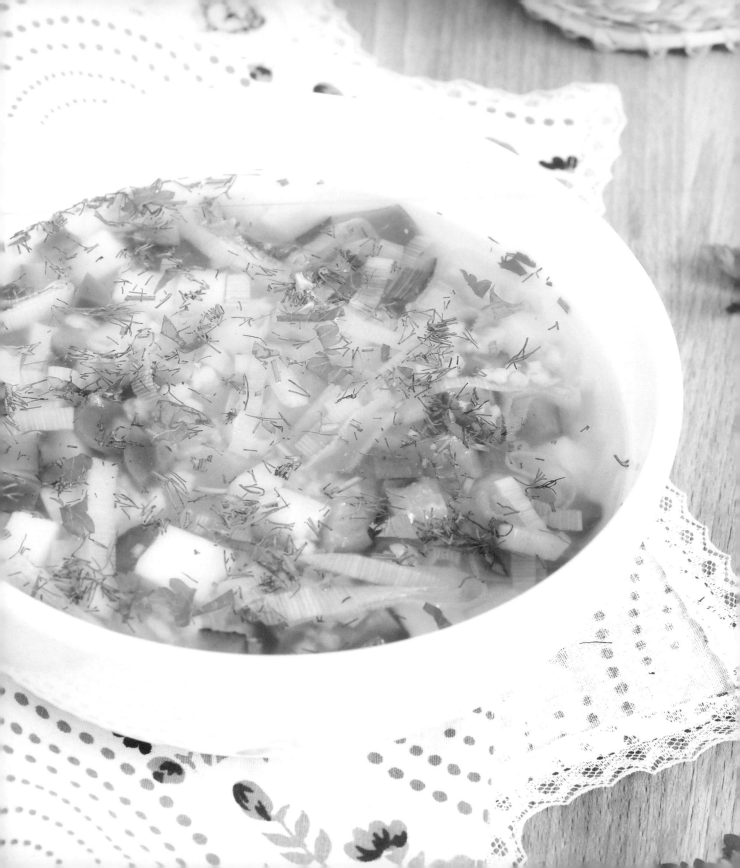

Chicken Soup with Fennel and Escarole

The licorice flavor of fresh fennel is reinforced by fennel seeds in this easy Italian healthful chicken soup.

Makes 4 to 6 servings.

1 pound boneless, skinless chicken breasts

1 large fennel bulb

3 tablespoons olive oil

2 large onions, diced

3 garlic cloves, minced

5 cups chicken stock or broth

1 14.5-oz can diced tomatoes, undrained

2 tcaspoons fennel seeds, crushed

1 head escarole

Salt and pepper to taste

1. Rinse the chicken and pat dry with paper towels. Trim chicken of all visible fat, and cut into ½-inch cubes. Rinse the fennel and cut in half lengthwise. Discard core and ribs, and dice bulb into ¾-inch pieces. Place the chicken and fennel in the slow cooker.

2. Heat olive oil in a medium skillet over medium-high heat. Add onions and garlic and cook, stirring frequently, until onions are translucent, about 3 minutes. Scrape mixture into slow cooker.

3. Stir stock, tomatoes (with juice), and fennel seeds into the slow cooker and stir to combine all ingredients. Cover and cook on Low for 5 to 7 hours or on High for 2½ to 3 hours, or until chicken is cooked through and tender. While soup cooks, rinse escarole. Cut in half, discard core, and cut the remaining escarole into 1-inch strips.

4. If cooking on Low, raise the heat to High. Add escarole to the slow cooker and cook for an additional 30 to 40 minutes, or until the escarole is wilted. Season to taste with salt and pepper, and serve hot.

Variation:

You can always substitute 2 celery ribs for each ½ fennel bulb specified in a recipe.

Fresh fennel, *finocchio* in Italian, and sometimes called anise in supermarkets, has a slightly licorice taste but the texture of celery—both raw and cooked.

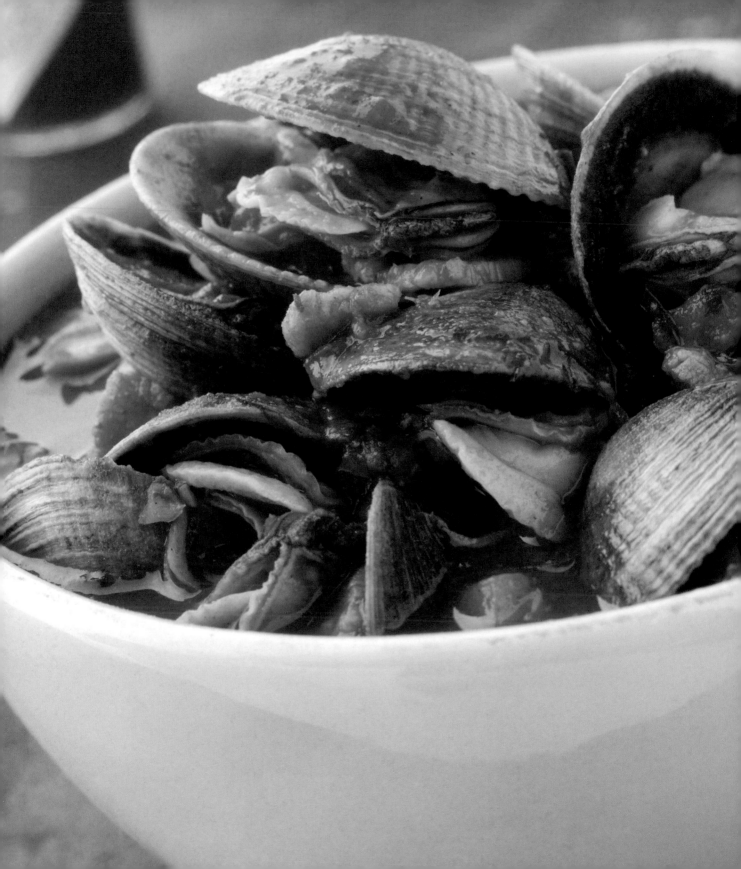

Zuppa de Arsella e Pancetta

The Adriatic coast is famous for its seafood dishes, and clams feature prominently in them. The pancetta in this recipe adds a touch of smokiness.

Makes 4 to 6 servings.

¼ pound pancetta, cut into 1-inch pieces

½ medium onion, diced

3 garlic cloves, minced

2 cups seafood stock or fish broth

2 tablespoons chopped fresh parsley

3 dozen fresh littleneck clams in the shell, the smallest ones

1. Cook pancetta pieces in a heavy skillet over medium-high heat for 5 to 7 minutes, or until crisp. Remove from the pan with a slotted spoon and drain on a plate covered with a paper towel. Discard all but 2 tablespoons of the grease. Add onions and garlic to the skillet and cook, stirring frequently, for about 3 minutes or until the onion is translucent. Turn off the heat, add the cooked pancetta, and stir to combine. Transfer the mixture to the slow cooker.

2. Add the seafood stock and parsley, and stir with the meat and onion mixture. Cover and cook on Low for 6 to 8 hours or on High for 3 to 4 hours.

3. At the end of the cooking time, prepare the clams. Soak them in a bowl of cold water for about 5 minutes. Fill a large bowl with cold water and, under cold running water, scrub each individual clam if it is sandy or gritty. Put the cleaned clams in the bowl of water until all are cleaned. If cooking on Low, raise the heat to High. Add the clams, cover and cook for another 30 minutes or so until the clams have opened. Place the opened clams into bowls, and ladle the seasoned stock over them.

Variations:
* You can make this soup without the pancetta if you want just the taste of the fresh clams.
* You can also substitute thick-cut bacon or a couple of links of Italian sausage, cut into bits. Hot Italian sausage complements the flavors very nicely.

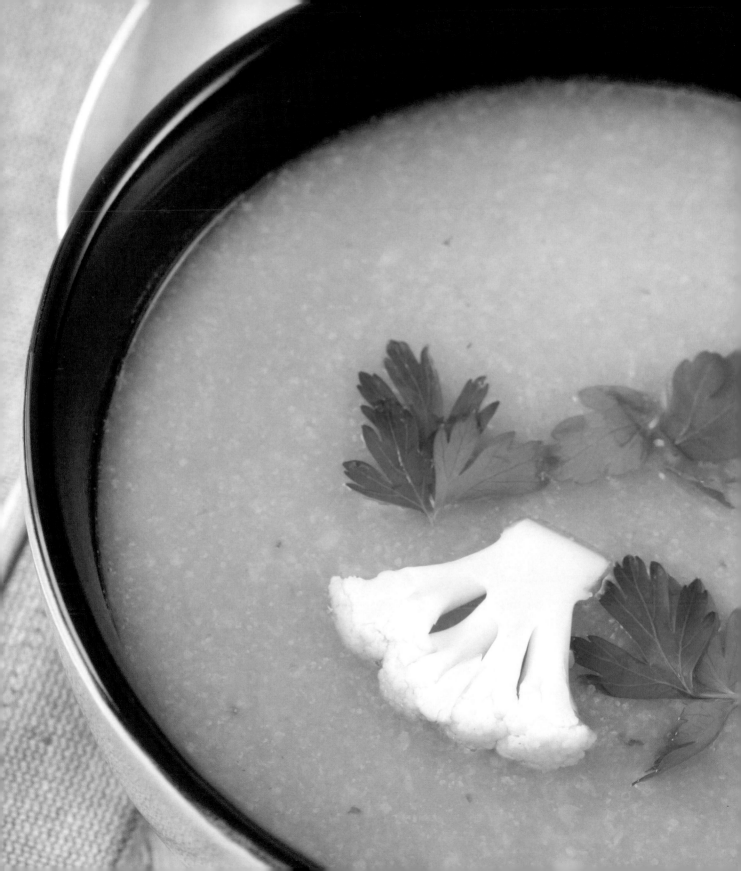

Creamy Cauliflower Soup

The nutty flavor of cauliflower shines through in this decadently creamy recipe. If you can find orange cauliflower, it not only has great color but contains about 25% more Vitamin A.

Makes 4 to 6 servings.

3 tablespoons olive oil

1 onion, chopped

2 cloves garlic, minced

3 tablespoons coconut flour

1 can coconut milk

2 cups chicken stock or broth

1 head cauliflower, broken up into pieces, tough stem removed, and rinsed

Salt and pepper to taste

1. In a skillet over medium-high heat, place 1 tablespoon olive oil and add onions and garlic. Cook stirring constantly until onions are translucent, about 5 minutes. Scrape mixture into the slow cooker.

2. Add the remaining 2 tablespoons of olive oil to the pan, working over medium heat. When hot, add the coconut flour 1 tablespoon at a time, stirring constantly with a wooden spoon to prevent any lumps from forming. When the flour is all added to the oil, you should have a thick paste. Next, stir in the coconut milk a little at a time, also stirring constantly to prevent lumping. When the milk is mixed in, you should have a thick, creamy mixture.

3. Pour this into the slow cooker. Add the stock and stir, and then add the cauliflower florets into the mix.

4. Cover and cook on Low for 6 to 8 hours or on High for 4 to 5 hours. If desired, puree the soup with an immersion blender or by batches in a blender.

Cauliflower, called *cavolfiore* in Italian, is enjoyed all over Italy. It is descended from wild cabbage and was cultivated along the Mediterranean coastlines of Turkey and Italy. Full of B6 and Vitamin D, it's as nutritious as it is delicious and makes a great substitute for potatoes in a Paleo diet.

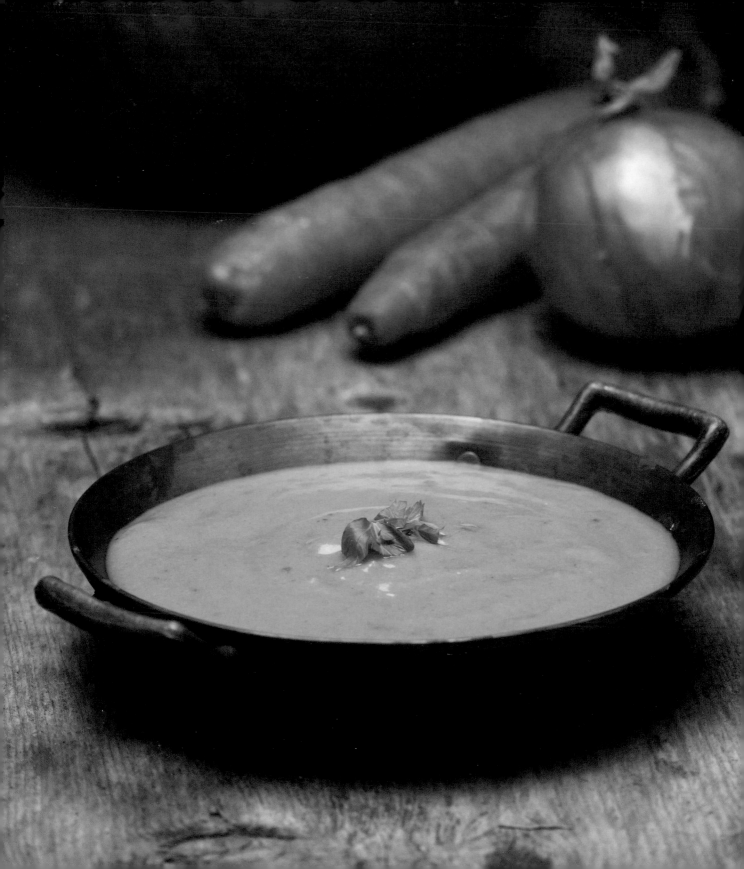

Pumpkin & Pear Soup

Italy is abundant in squashes, and pumpkin features in a lot of their dishes, whether on its own, in a soup or stew, or as a filling for pasta. This recipe is *multo bene* any time you make it.

Makes 6 servings.

2 tablespoons olive oil

1 large onion, chopped

2 pounds pumpkin (or butternut squash) peeled, seeded, and cut into 2-inch pieces

2 Bosc pears, peeled, cored and cubed

4 carrots, peeled and cut into thin slices

6 cups chicken broth

Sprigs of fresh thyme

6 fresh sage leaves

Salt to taste

1. Heat the oil in a skillet and add the onions, cooking over medium-high heat until translucent, about 3 to 5 minutes.

2. Combine the pumpkin, pears, and carrots in the slow cooker. Stir in the chicken broth. Add the cooked onions and stir. Put 3 thyme sprigs on top. Cover and cook on Low for 4 to 5 hours or on High for 2 to 3 hours or until vegetables and fruit are cooked through and soft. Remove the thyme sprigs.

3. Puree with an immersion blender or in batches in a food processor or blender. Season to taste with salt. Serve hot. Garnish with the sage leaves and some additional thyme if desired.

Variation:
You can substitute dried herbs for the fresh thyme and sage in this recipe, since they can be hard to come by in the winter. If you go this route, use 2 teaspoons dried thyme instead of the fresh sprigs, and stir in 1 teaspoon dried sage before serving the hot soup.

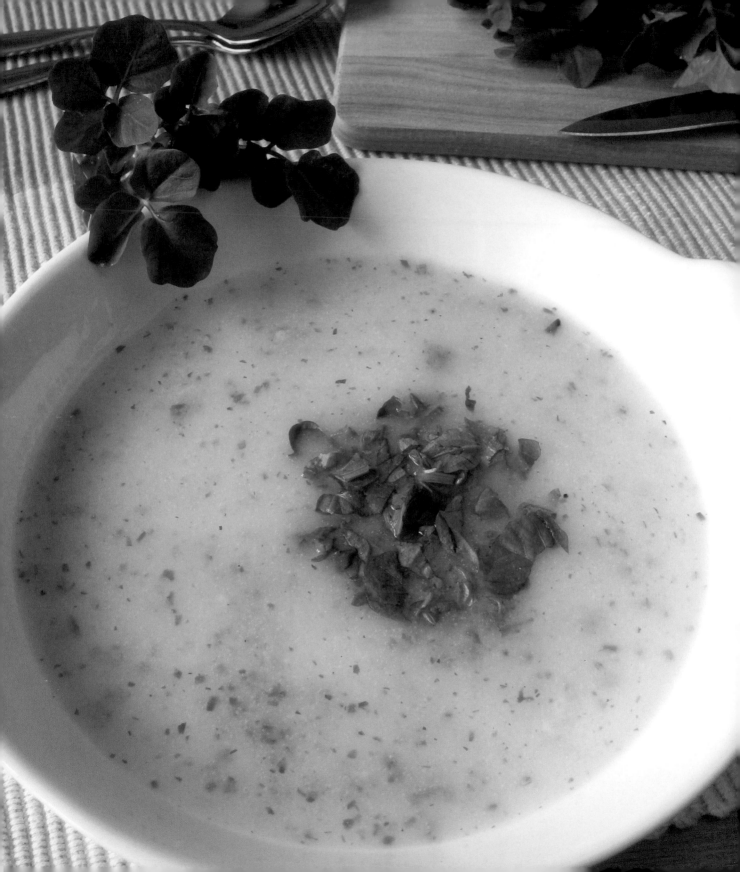

Watercress & Mushroom Soup

If you like the tangy yet delicate flavor of watercress, you will love this soup.

Makes 8 to 10 servings.

2 tablespoons olive oil

2 cloves garlic, minced

1 small zucchini, cut into small pieces

1 large Portobello mushroom, washed, patted dry, and chopped

2 bunches watercress, washed, dried, and some stalk removed

8 cups chicken broth

Salt and pepper to taste

1. In a large saucepan over medium heat, add the olive oil. When hot, add the garlic and cook, stirring, for a minute or so. Don't let the garlic burn. Add the zucchini and mushroom pieces and stir. Cook the vegetables for about 5 minutes. Transfer the mixture into the slow cooker.

2. Add the watercress and stir. Pour the chicken broth over all the vegetables. Cover and cook on Low for 5 to 6 hours or on High for 3 to 4 hours until all vegetables are tender.

3. Serve chunky, or process to a liquid with an immersion blender or in a food processor. Season with salt and pepper.

> Watercress is believed to be one of the oldest leafy vegetables consumed by humans, so it's a super Paleo food! It's full of vitamins and minerals. Its delicate leaves pack a punch in nutrition and flavor.

Variation:

If watercress is too tangy for you, try spinach.

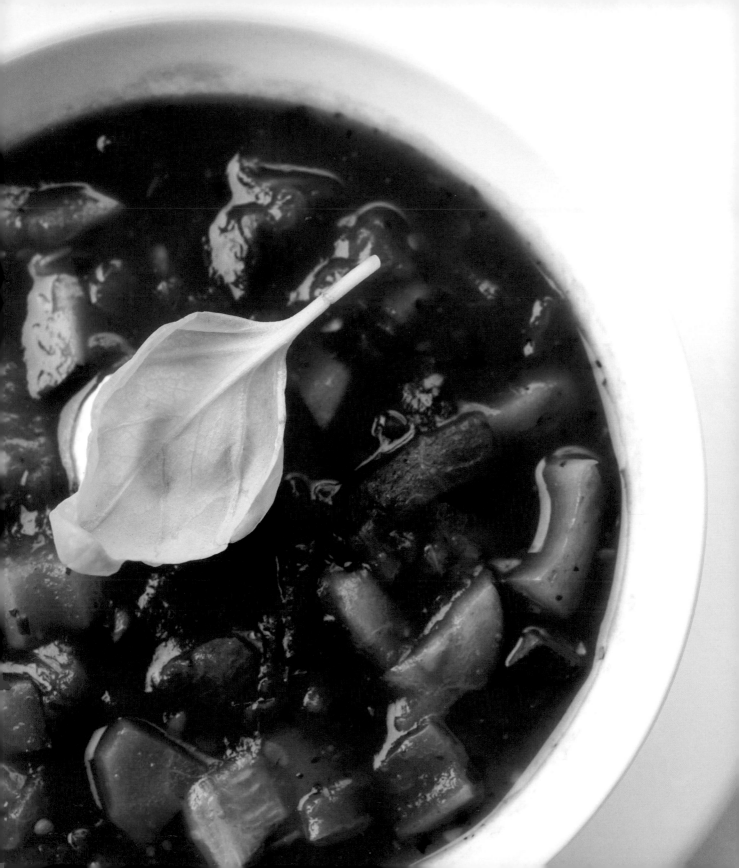

Classic Minestrone

In Italy, *minestrone* is synonymous with vegetable soup. It can be made many ways—with or without meat, for example—and usually includes vegetables that are in season. It dates back to ancient times and typically includes beans. This Paleo-friendly recipe excludes the beans but takes advantage of fresh vegetables.

Makes 6 to 8 servings.

2 tablespoons olive oil

1 onion, chopped

2 cloves garlic, chopped

4 cups vegetable stock

2 (14.5 ounce) cans stewed tomatoes

2 stalks celery, chopped

2 carrots, sliced

1 large head cabbage, finely chopped

2 small, thin zucchini, sliced

½ teaspoon dried oregano

¼ teaspoon dried thyme

salt and pepper to taste

1. Heat the oil in a saucepan over medium heat. Add the onions and garlic and cook, stirring, until the onions are just slightly translucent, about two minutes.

2. Transfer the onion/garlic mix to the slow cooker. Add the vegetable stock, undrained tomatoes, celery, carrots, cabbage, and zucchini. Cook on Low for 5 to 7 hours or on High for 2 to 3 hours, until vegetables are tender. Stir in seasonings, and allow to cook for an additional 15 minutes. Serve hot.

Variations:

If you'd like to add meat to this soup, there are several tasty options.

✻ One is to slice a couple of sausages and sauté them with the onions and garlic.

✻ Another is to add diced cooked chicken when you add the seasonings in the last part of the cooking.

✻ Still another is to make a dozen or so mini meatballs with ½ pound ground turkey mixed with 1 tablespoon chopped fresh parsley and put them into the vegetable and broth mixture just before starting the cooking. If you do that, extend the cooking time on Low by about 1 hour and on High for 15 to 20 minutes.

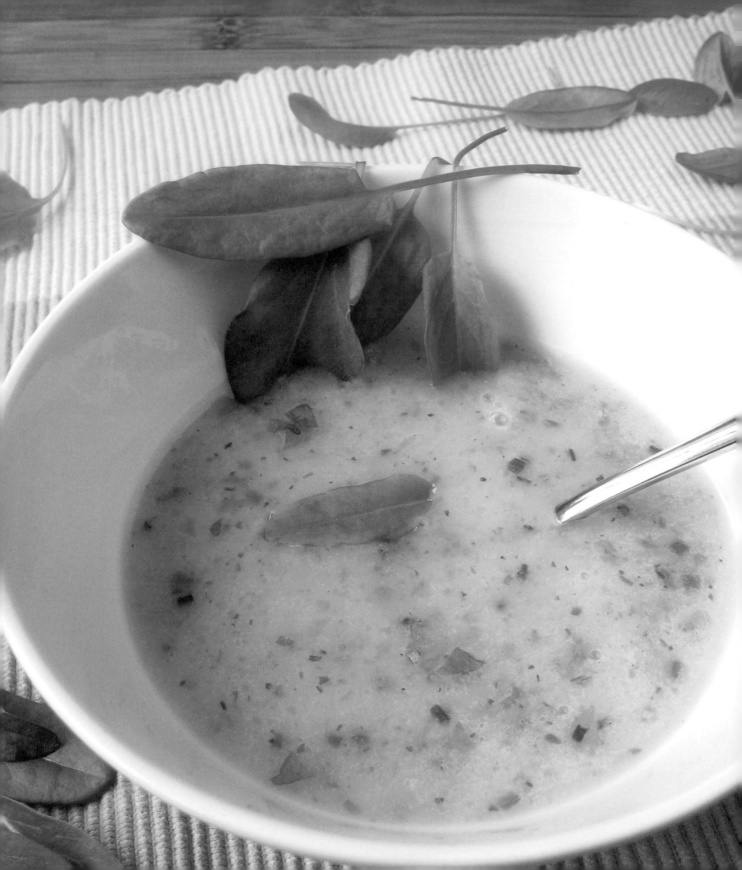

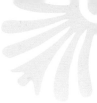

Spring Sorrel Soup

Sorrel is actually a large herb but is harvested as a leafy vegetable. It has a distinct lemon-tart flavor that makes an excellent soup—especially with the addition of the coconut milk.

Makes 4 to 6 servings.

1 tablespoon olive oil

1 onion, chopped

2 cups chicken broth

1½ cups coconut milk

2 cups fresh sorrel, stems removed and coarsely chopped

Salt and pepper to taste

1. Heat the olive oil in a skillet and add onions, cooking until translucent, about 5 minutes.

2. Transfer mixture to the slow cooker. Add the chicken broth and coconut milk. Cover and cook on Low for 4 to 5 hours or on High for 2 to 3 hours.

3. Add the sorrel. Cook an additional hour on Low and 30 minutes on High. Process with an immersion blender or food processer and season with salt and pepper.

You're not likely to find sorrel in the supermarket, but at a good farmer's market you should find it in the spring. It's easy to grow and is common across Europe. It is high in Vitamin C. The characteristic tartness is from the oxalic acid in the leaves, which is more pronounced in larger, older leaves. Younger leaves are great to put in salad.

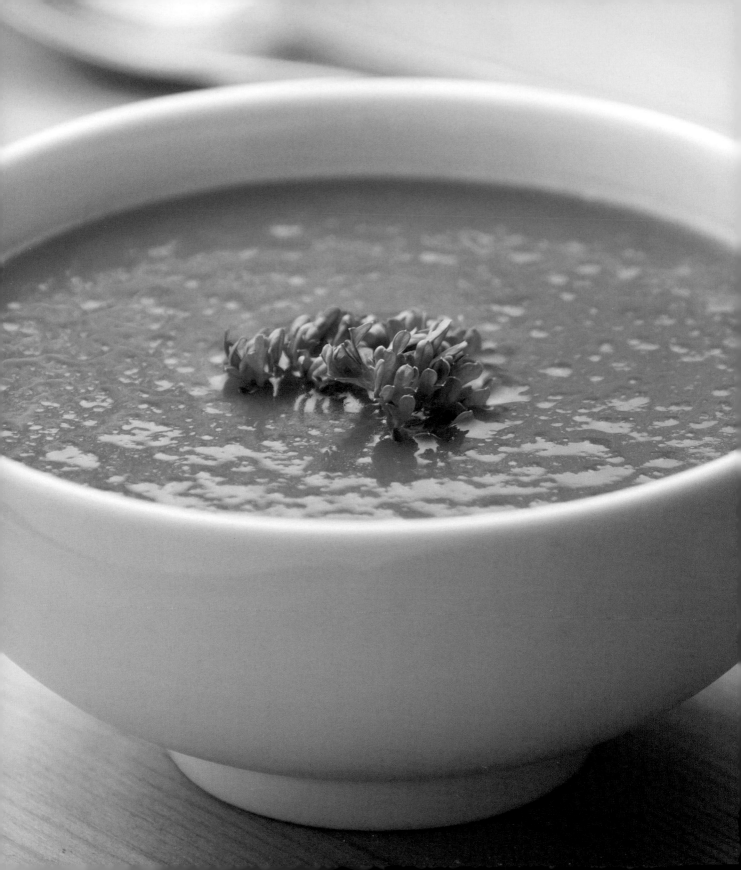

Tomato Soup

For the ultimate flavor, make this soup when tomatoes are at their ripest—late summer. If you want a creamy soup, add some coconut milk when pureeing the solids.

Makes 4 to 6 servings.

3 tablespoons olive oil

1 onion, diced

2 fresh anchovy filets

4 pounds ripe tomatoes, seeds removed and chopped

2 cups chicken stock or broth

½ to ¾ cup coconut milk, if desired

Ground black pepper to taste

1. In a skillet over medium-high heat, add the oil and onion. Cook the onion until translucent, about 5 minutes. Lower the heat and add the anchovy filets, mashing them into the onion and oil mixture until they are crushed. Scrape mixture into the slow cooker.

2. Add the tomatoes and stock. Cover and cook on Low for 6 to 8 hours or on high for 4 to 5 hours.

3. Puree the soup using an immersion blender. If you want to make the soup creamy, add the coconut milk while you're pureeing it. Season with freshly ground pepper; the anchovies provide the saltiness.

Variation:
Garnish with a "bruschetta" of finely chopped tomatoes, cucumbers, and parsley for added color, flavor, and nutrition.

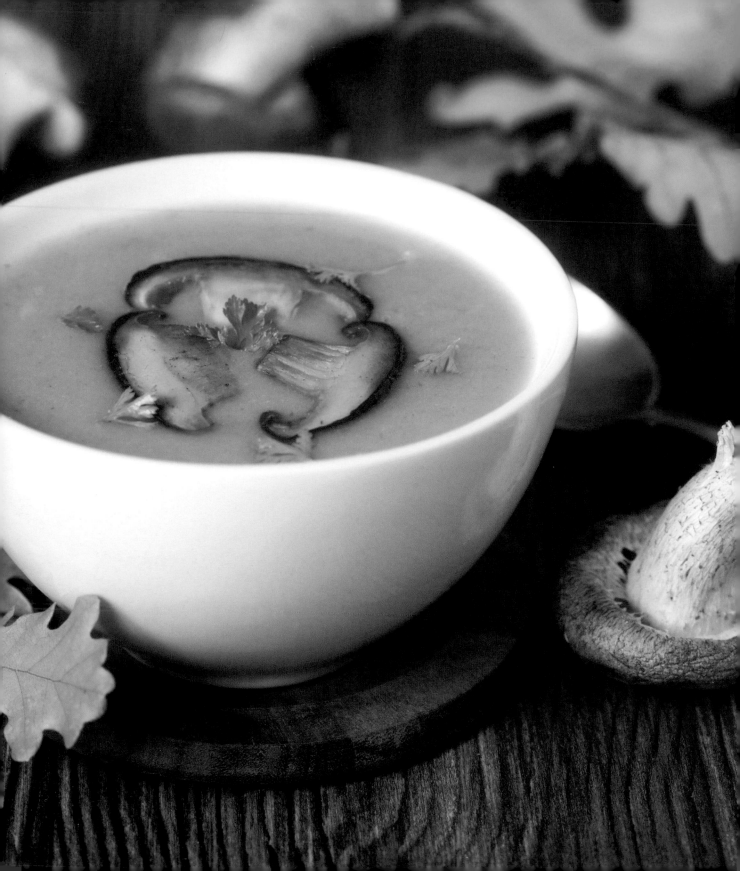

Mushroom Bisque

An earthy, rich, mushroom bisque—like this one laced with sherry—will get any evening off to a festive start, whether you're serving it at a more formal gathering or sharing a bowl with a friend by the fire.

Makes 4 to 6 servings.

1 cup dried wild mushrooms, like chanterelles or porcini

1 tablespoon olive oil

1 tablespoon ghee

½ onion, diced fine

1 stalk celery, thinly sliced

2 pounds fresh mushrooms, such as button or shiitake

1 teaspoon fresh rosemary leaves, chopped

¼ cup sweet sherry

1 cup chicken broth or stock

1 teaspoon fresh tarragon leaves, chopped

Salt and pepper to taste

1. Bring about 2 cups of water to a boil. Place dried mushrooms in a large glass bowl or measuring cup. Pour the boiling water over the mushrooms and set aside. Tap or gently rinse the dirt off the fresh mushrooms, cut into small pieces, and set aside.

2. Heat oil and ghee in a large skillet over medium heat. Add onions and cook, stirring occasionally, until onions are translucent, about 3 minutes. Add the celery, fresh mushrooms, and rosemary, and continue to cook a couple of more minutes. Transfer the mixture to the slow cooker. Add the sherry and porcinis with their broth. Cover and cook on Low for 3 to 4 hours or on High for about 2 hours. Add tarragon in the last hour of cooking.

3. Using a standard or immersion blender, puree soup until smooth. If using a standard blender, puree in small batches to prevent spillage. Season with salt and pepper.

Mushrooms are called *funghi* in Italy, and they are everywhere, which is great for people who love their comforting, earthy flavor. This soup truly warms the body and soul.

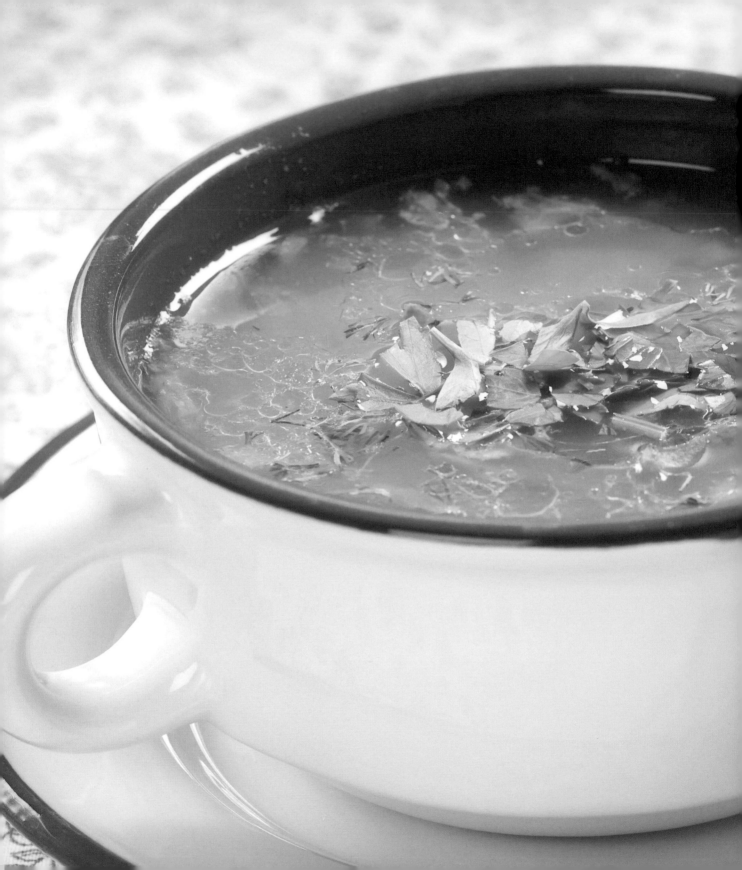

Cabbage and Carrot Soup

You'll find the carrots mellow the cabbage in this soup with a beautiful flavor and texture. And it's loaded with healthy veggies.

Makes 4 servings.

4 tablespoons olive oil

1 large onion, chopped

1 pound green cabbage, sliced thin and washed

2 small zucchini, washed and sliced thin

2 carrots, peeled and sliced thin

1 apple, peeled and sliced thin

4 cups chicken broth

1 tablespoon fresh rosemary, minced

Salt to taste

1. Heat the oil in a skillet and add the onion. Cook over medium-high heat until onions are translucent, about 3 minutes.

2. Put the cabbage, zucchini, carrots, apple, and cooked onion in the slow cooker. Add the chicken broth, cover, and cook on Low for 3 to 4 hours or on High for 2 to 3 hours. Check the soup. The cabbage should be cooked but still fairly firm. When it's cooked and ready to serve, stir in the rosemary. Season to taste with salt and serve.

This is a delicious soup made from vegetables that overwinter well. The rosemary is the Italian touch, and you could also squeeze in a spritz of lemon before serving.

Variation:
Consider varying the ingredients by substituting similar veggies, like squash, broccoli, Brussels sprouts, and so on.

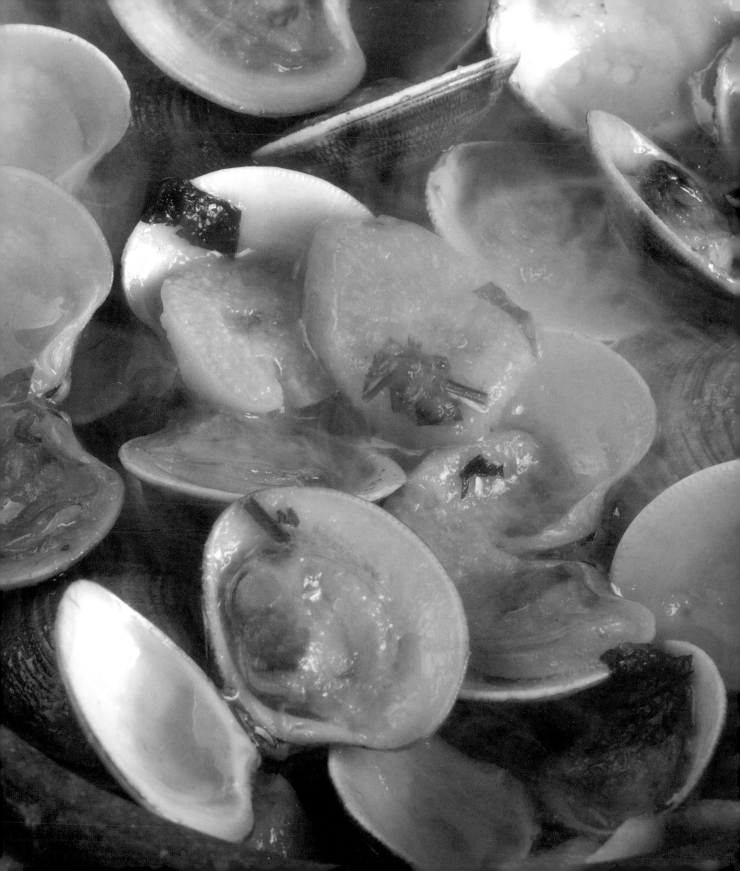

Vegetable Soup with Clams

This soup is like an Italian version of Manhattan clam chowder. In Italy it's served with tiny whole clams, but the minced clams are easier to eat with the rest of the soup.

Makes 4 to 6 servings.

1 pint minced fresh clams

2 tablespoons olive oil

2 fresh anchovy filets, finely chopped

1 small onion, diced

2 cloves garlic, minced

1 celery rib, diced

1 carrot, chopped fine

½ green bell pepper, seeds and ribs removed, and chopped

1 cup butternut squash or pumpkin, peeled and cubed

1 14.5-ounce can crushed tomatoes, undrained

1 8-ounce bottle clam juice

1 cup dry white wine

1 tablespoon capers, drained and rinsed

3 tablespoons fresh parsley, chopped

1 tablespoon fresh thyme

½ teaspoon dried oregano

2 bay leaves

Salt and pepper to taste

1. Drain clams, reserving juice. Refrigerate clams until ready to serve.

2. Heat oil in a medium skillet over medium heat. Add anchovies, onion, garlic, celery, carrot, and green bell pepper. Cook, stirring frequently, for 3 minutes, or until onion is translucent. Scrape mixture into the slow cooker.

3. Add squash, tomatoes, clam juice, wine, capers, juice drained from clams, parsley, thyme, oregano, and bay leaves to the slow cooker, and stir well. Cook on Low for 5 to 7 hours or on High for 2½ to 3 hours, or until squash is almost tender.

4. If cooking on Low, raise the heat to High. Add clams, and continue to cook for an additional 20 to 40 minutes, or until clams are cooked through. Remove and discard bay leaves, season to taste with salt and pepper, and serve hot.

It's now possible to find fresh minced clams in just about every supermarket. If they're not in the refrigerated case, check the freezer. If you must resort to canned clams, use 3 (6-ounce) cans for each pint of fresh clams specified.

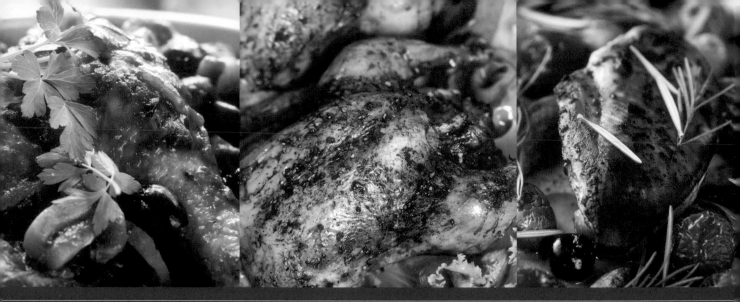

Chapter 5

Paleo *Secondi:*
Poultry and Duck

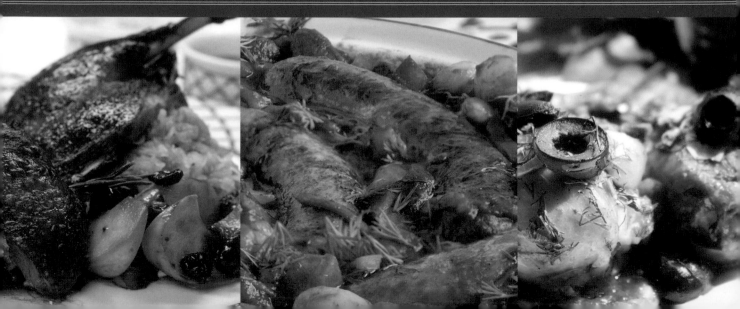

*I*talian vegetables, herbs, and even nuts combine beautifully with the mild flavors of chicken or turkey, as well as the more earthy and robust flavor of duck. Other ingredients that enliven Italian poultry and duck dishes and that are Paleo-friendly and plentiful in the recipes in this chapter are olives, mushrooms, peppers, leeks, fruits, and truffle oil. The beauty, again, is that there are seasonal ingredients you can find and use in combination to create delicious, healthy, and easy-to-make poultry *secondi* any time of the year.

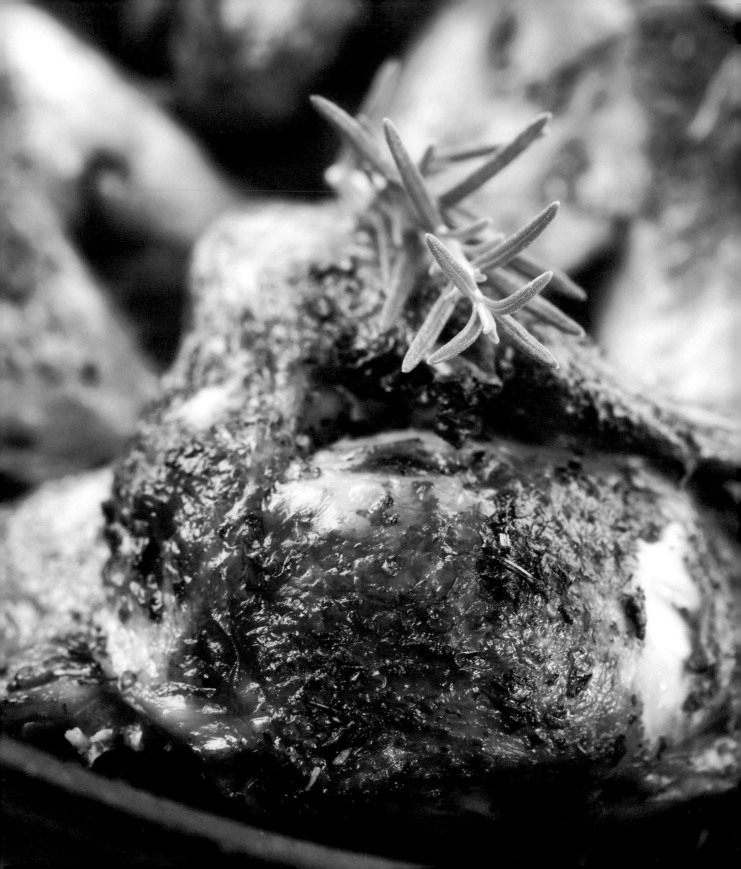

Sensational Roast Chicken

The slow cooking yields tender, fragrant meat. If you want crisp skin, put the cooked chicken under the broiler in the oven for about 5 minutes. Chances are it won't matter to you when this is done.

Makes 6 to 8 servings.

1 onion, cut into thick slivers
1 carrot, sliced
1 4- to 5-lb whole chicken
1 lemon
1 teaspoon dried thyme
1 teaspoon dried sage
1 teaspoon sea salt
1 teaspoon ground black pepper
Fresh rosemary for garnish

1. Place the slivers of onion and the sliced carrot in the slow cooker. Put the chicken on top of the vegetables. Squeeze the lemon over everything, then slice it into rounds and put a couple of the slices in the cavity of the bird. Season all over with thyme, sage, salt, and pepper.

2. Cover and cook on Low for 6 to 8 hours or on High for 3 to 4 hours. Season with additional salt and pepper. Garnish with rosemary.

You could substitute an already-made blend of spices called Poultry Seasoning for the thyme and sage. The poultry blend contains those herbs, as well as marjoram, parsley, and sometimes savory and rosemary.

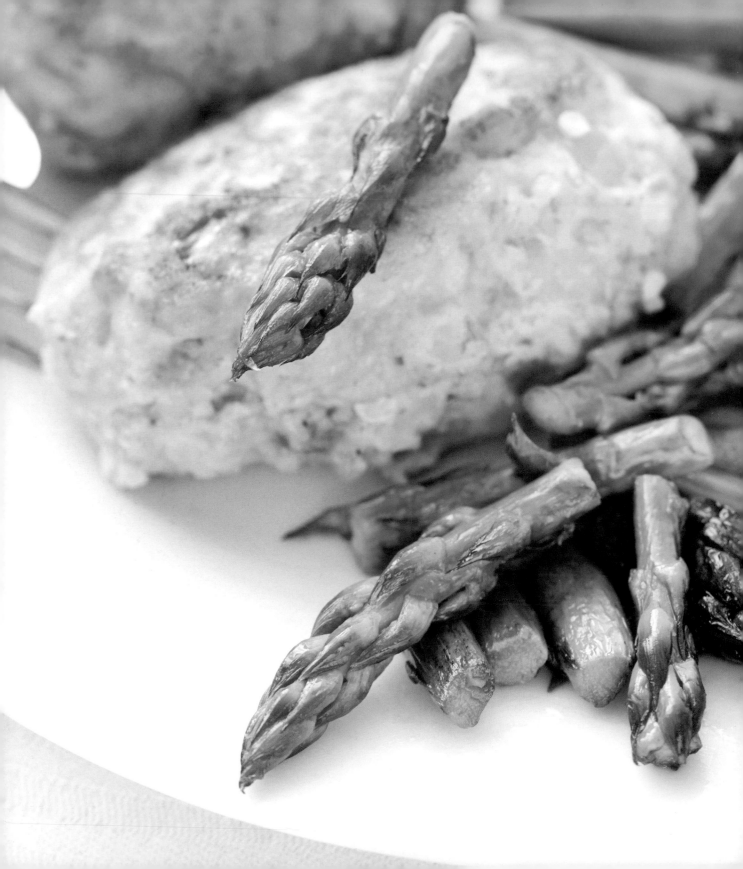

Chicken with Spring Vegetables

Chicken is inherently delicate, and that quality is conveyed beautifully in this light dish with accents of pearl onion, asparagus, and even Bibb lettuce.

Makes 4 to 6 servings.

6 chicken thighs, skin removed

2 cups chicken stock or broth

3 tablespoons fresh parsley, chopped

1 tablespoon fresh thyme

1 tablespoon fresh rosemary, chopped

1 tablespoon fresh tarragon

1 bay leaf

2 cloves garlic, minced

1 10-oz package frozen pearl onions, thawed

6 stalks asparagus, tough bottoms removed, cut into ½-inch pieces

2 heads Bibb lettuce, trimmed and cut into quarters

Salt and pepper to taste

1. Rinse chicken and pat dry with paper towels. Preheat the oven broiler, and line a broiler pan with heavy-duty aluminum foil. Broil chicken pieces for 3 minutes per side, or until browned.

2. Add stock, parsley, thyme, rosemary, tarragon, bay leaf, garlic, pearl onions, and asparagus pieces to the cooker, and stir well. Arrange chicken pieces in the slow cooker, and cook on Low for 5 to 7 hours or on High for 2 to 3 hours, or until chicken is almost cooked through.

3. If cooking on Low, raise the heat to High. Add lettuce, and cook for another 30 minutes, or until lettuce is wilted, chicken is tender, and mixture is bubbling. Remove and discard bay leaf, and season to taste with salt and pepper.

Variation:

Other spring vegetables you could add include a handful or so of young dandelion leaves or ramps, which are wild leeks (in the onion family). These tender vegetables should be added toward the end of the cooking time, as with the lettuce in the recipe.

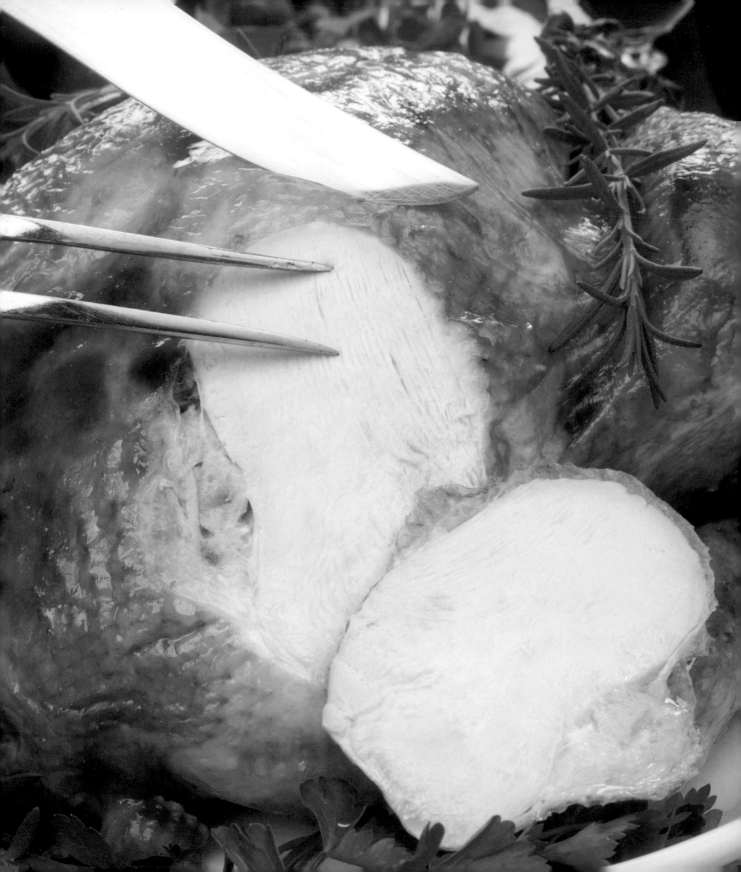

Turkey Breast with Rosemary

You might find yourself preparing this at the end of every week so you can slice into it as your week gets busy. It makes a lovely, finished meat that can be used to top salads, roll in lettuce leaves, or even eat out of the fridge.

Makes 4 to 6 servings.

4-pound boneless, skinless turkey breast
½ teaspoon salt
¼ teaspoon pepper
1 tablespoon fresh rosemary, chopped
1 tablespoon fresh parsley, chopped
½ cup chicken stock or broth

1. Place the turkey in the slow cooker. Sprinkle with salt and pepper, add herbs, and add stock.

2. Cover and cook on Low for 7 to 9 hours or on High for 4 to 6 hours, or until the meat is cooked through.

Variation:
For easy-to-make, healthy, and delicious snacks, put cut cooked turkey onto a Romaine lettuce leaf, and top with roasted peppers, thinly sliced onions, tomatoes, and/or slivered almonds. Roll the filling up in the leaf and enjoy.

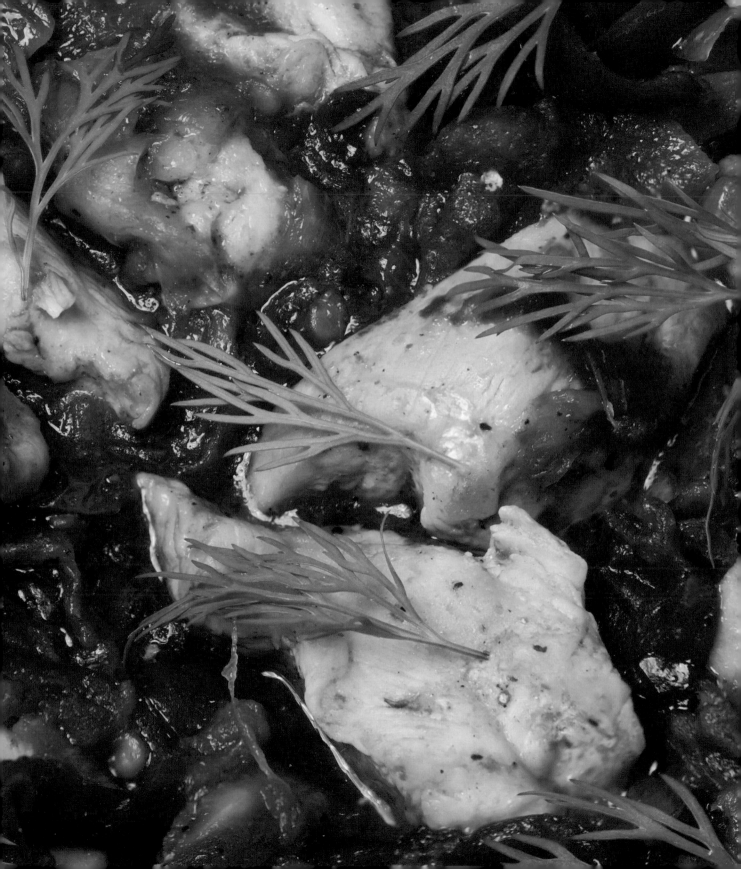

Chicken with Peppers

This dish of chicken cooked with sweet bell peppers and herbs in red wine comes from Umbria, Italy. Prepared in the slow cooker, it brings the melded flavors of the meat and the peppers together *con gusto!* Serve over spaghetti squash.

Makes 4 to 6 servings.

6 chicken pieces, skin removed

3 tablespoons olive oil

2 onions, diced

3 cloves garlic, minced

1 carrot, diced

1 rib celery, diced

3 red bell peppers, seeds and ribs removed, cut into thin strips

1 cup dry white wine

14.5-oz can diced tomatoes, undrained

1 tablespoon orange zest

3 tablespoons fresh parsley, chopped

2 tablespoons fresh oregano

1 tablespoon tomato paste

Salt and pepper to taste

1. Rinse chicken and pat dry with paper towels. Preheat the oven broiler, and line a broiler pan with heavy-duty aluminum foil. Broil chicken pieces for 3 minutes per side, or until browned. Transfer to the slow cooker.

2. Heat oil in a large skillet over medium-high heat. Add onion, garlic, carrot, celery, and red bell pepper. Cook, stirring frequently, for 5 minutes, or until pepper begins to soften.

3. Add wine, tomatoes, orange zest, parsley, oregano, and tomato paste to the cooker, and stir well to dissolve tomato paste. Cook on Low for 6 to 8 hours or on High for 3 to 4 hours, or until chicken is cooked through, tender, and no longer pink. Season to taste with salt and pepper.

Variation:

Save the flavored oil in an airtight container and use it in place of olive or coconut oil to flavor sauteed onions or other sauteed veggies, or drizzle it over cooked meat or eggs.

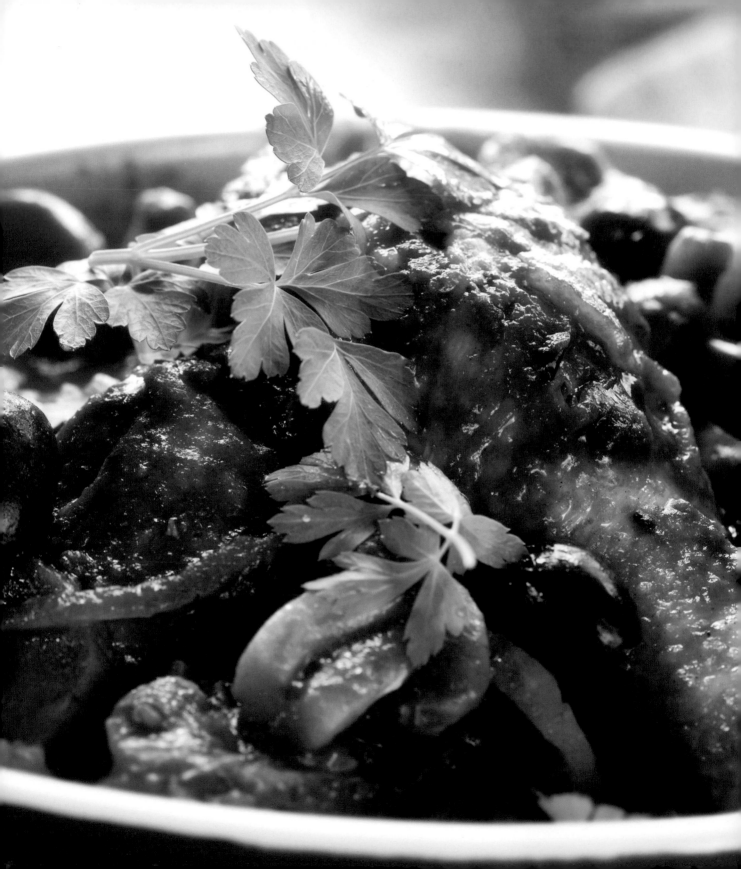

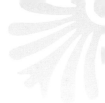

Chicken with Mushrooms

Cacciatore is Italian for "hunter's style," and Italians in all regions are hunters. Though several meats can be featured in a cacciatore, they all include tomatoes, onions, pancetta, and mushrooms.

Makes 4 to 6 servings.

6 chicken pieces, skin removed

¼ cup olive oil

2 large onions, halved and thinly sliced

2 cloves garlic, minced

1 pound cremini mushrooms, wiped with a damp paper towel, trimmed, and sliced

1 28-oz can diced tomatoes, undrained

½ cup dry white wine

1 tablespoon fresh thyme

1 tablespoon fresh sage, chopped

1 tablespoon fresh rosemary, chopped

Salt and pepper to taste

1. Rinse chicken and pat dry with paper towels. Preheat the oven broiler, and line a broiler pan with heavy-duty aluminum foil. Broil chicken pieces for 3 minutes per side, or until browned. Transfer pieces to the slow cooker.

2. Heat oil in a large skillet over medium-high heat. Add onions, garlic, and mushrooms and cook, stirring frequently, for 5 minutes, or until mushrooms begin to soften. Scrape mixture into the slow cooker.

3. Add tomatoes, wine, thyme, sage, and rosemary to the cooker, and stir well. Cook on Low for 6 to 8 hours or on High for 3 to 4 hours, or until chicken is cooked through, tender, and no longer pink. Season to taste with salt and pepper.

> Most of the mushrooms we find in supermarkets are the same species, *Agaricus bisporus*. What makes the difference is their age. White button mushrooms are the youngest, cremini are in the middle, and Portobello is what we call them when they're big and older.

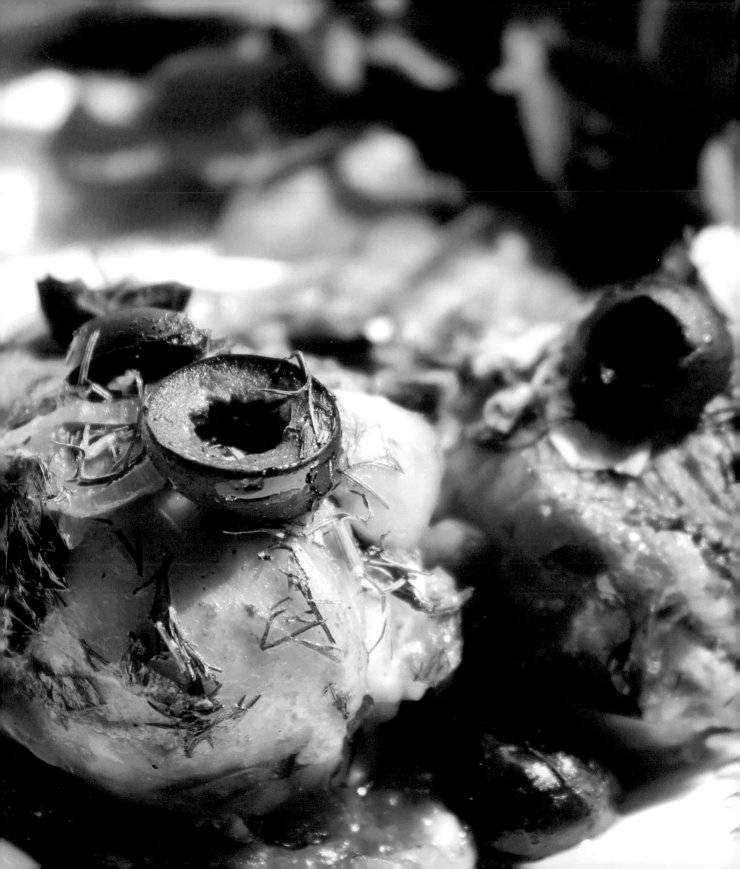

Chicken with Peppers and Olives

Both oranges and olives grow all over Sicily, and those are joined by colorful bell peppers in this exuberant dish that will have you thinking you're vacationing in *la bella Italia!*

Makes 4 to 6 servings.

6 chicken pieces, skin removed

¼ cup olive oil

1 large onions, diced

2 cloves garlic, minced

1 green bell pepper, seeds and ribs removed, diced

1 red bell pepper, seeds and ribs removed, diced

½ cup freshly squeezed orange juice

½ cup chicken stock or broth

½ cup dry white wine

1 14.5-oz can diced tomatoes, undrained

1 tablespoon fresh thyme

1 tablespoon fresh rosemary, chopped

1 tablespoon grated orange zest

2 bay leaves

½ cup pitted oil-cured black olives

Salt and pepper to taste

1. Rinse chicken and pat dry with paper towels. Preheat the oven broiler, and line a broiler pan with heavy-duty aluminum foil. Broil chicken pieces for 3 minutes per side, or until browned. Transfer pieces to the slow cooker.

2. Heat oil in a large skillet over medium-high heat. Add onions, garlic, green pepper, and red pepper. Cook, stirring frequently, for 5 minutes, or until onion is translucent. Scrape mixture into the slow cooker.

3. Add orange juice, stock, wine, tomatoes, parsley, thyme, rosemary, orange zest, bay leaves, and olives to the cooker, and stir well. Cook on Low for 6 to 8 hours or on High for 3 to 4 hours, or until chicken is cooked through, tender, and no longer pink. Remove and discard bay leaves. Season to taste with salt and pepper.

Crispy skin doesn't happen when you're cooking chicken in the slow cooker. That's just a fact. While the chicken is browned for all of these recipes so that the skin looks appealing and not pasty white, if you want crisp skin, place the pieces under the oven broiler, about 8 inches beneath the element, for 3 to 5 minutes, and the skin will become crisp.

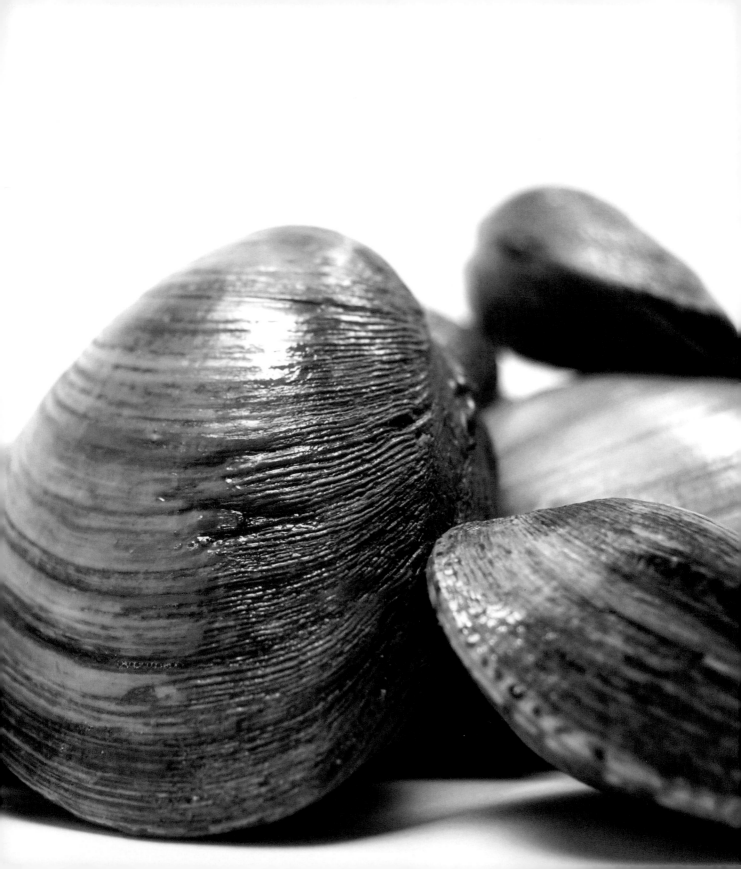

Chicken and Clams

This is a "surf and turf" indulgence that'll have you coming back for more.

Makes 4 to 6 servings.

2 tablespoons olive oil

½ cup of almond flour

Salt for seasoning the almond flour

6 pieces of chicken, bone in and skinless

1 medium carrot, peeled and sliced

1 tablespoon fresh ginger, peeled and minced

1 medium white onion, diced

½ cup water

2 dozen littleneck clams, rinsed in several changes of water until water runs clear, and drained

½ cup fresh parsley, chopped

1. Heat the oil over medium-high heat in a large skillet. Put the flour in a pie plate or shallow bowl and season it with salt. Coat the chicken pieces with the flour, shaking off any excess, and put on a plate. When the oil is hot, put the chicken pieces in it. Cook the chicken, turning every so often, until the chicken is browned on all sides.

2. Put the chicken pieces in the slow cooker. Add the carrot, ginger, onion, and water. Cover and cook on low for 4 to 5 hours.

3. Turn the heat to high so that the liquid is bubbling. Add the clams, replace the cover, and cook an additional 30 to 40 minutes, or until the clams are opened. Garnish with fresh parsley.

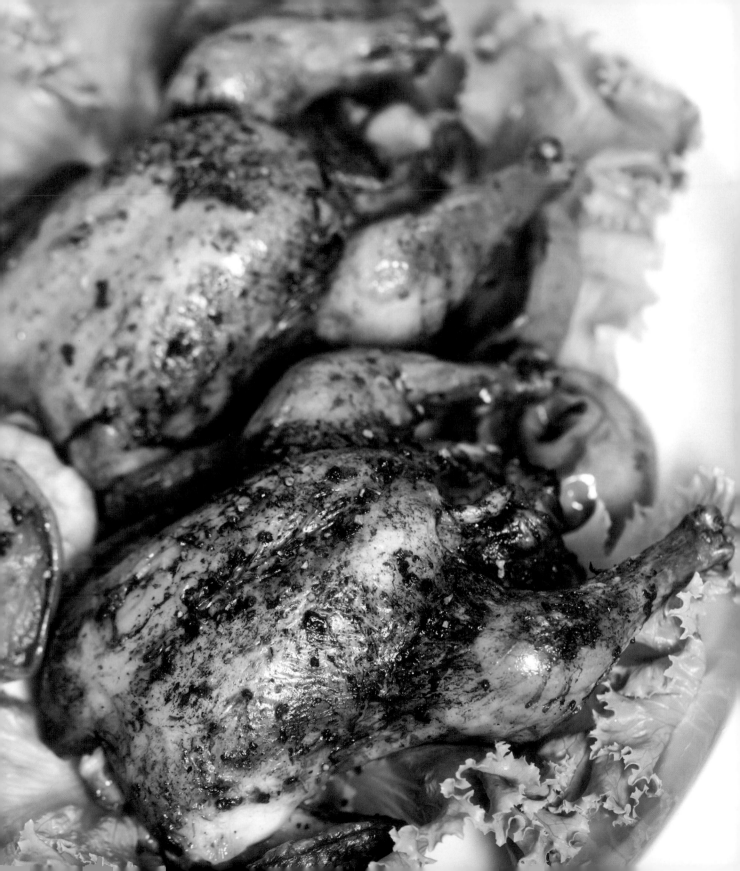

Cornish Hens with Fresh Greens

Cornish hens are as easy to make as dishes with chicken pieces, but there's something about them that makes the meal seem extra-special.

Makes 4 to 6 servings.

2 tablespoons olive oil

1 small onion, minced

1 garlic clove, minced

2 small Cornish game hens, split in two, skin removed

1 head Swiss chard, washed, coarse stems removed, and leaves chopped in large pieces

1 head Escarole, washed, trimmed, and chopped in large pieces

½ cup chicken stock or broth

1 pound baby spinach leaves

Salt and pepper to taste

1. Heat oil in a small skillet over medium-high heat, and cook onions and garlic about 3 minutes, or until onion is translucent. Scrape mixture into slow cooker.

2. Place Cornish hens on top of onion mixture, and top with Swiss chard, Escarole, and broth.

3. Cover the slow cooker and cook on Low for 6 to 7 hours or on High for 3 to 4 hours, or until chicken is tender and cooked through. Add the baby spinach and cook for another 20 to 30 minutes. Season with salt and pepper.

The Cornish Game hen is a young, immature chicken, which is technically not supposed to be over 5 weeks of age or more than 2 pounds. It's the result of crossing the Cornish Game and Plymouth or White Rock chicken breeds. For Paleo purposes, you probably won't find these at farmer's markets, so they won't be as fresh as free-range birds. But they are impressive and a nice change of pace.

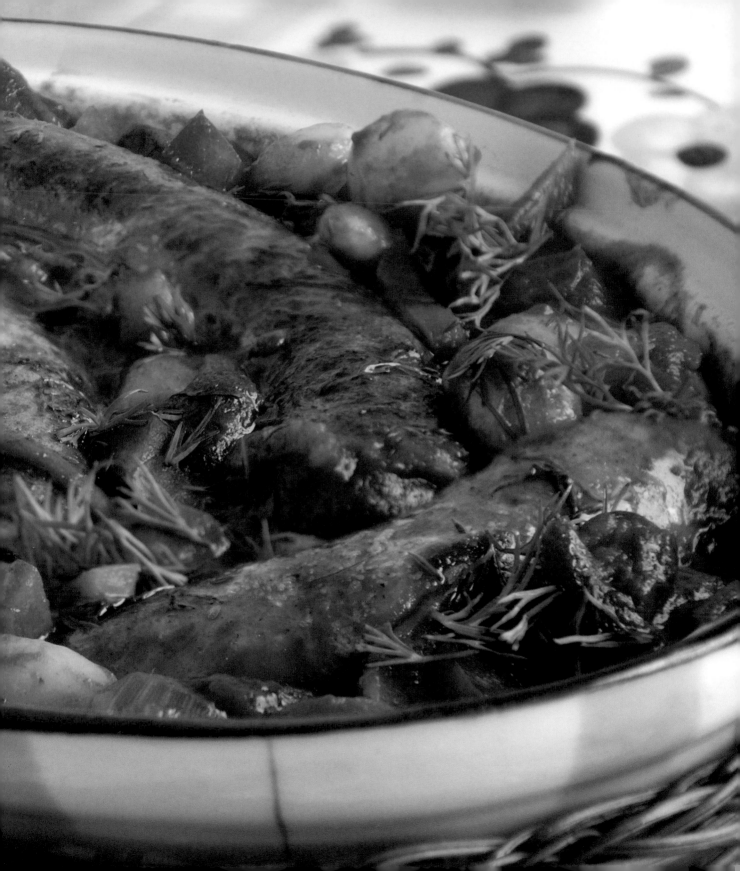

Pheasant and Sausage Stew

This stew is a hearty and flavorful dish, with both sausage and pancetta enlivening the flavor. Serve with a salad of tangy greens, like arugula.

Makes 4 to 6 servings.

2 pounds pheasant pieces

2 juice oranges, washed

¼ pound pancetta or bacon, diced

1 medium onion, diced

1 carrot, sliced

1 celery rib, sliced

3 cloves garlic, minced

½ pound fresh pork sausage

1 14.5-oz can diced tomatoes, undrained

3½ cups chicken stock or broth

3 tablespoons fresh basil, chopped

2 tablespoons fresh parsley, chopped

1 tablespoon fresh thyme, chopped

1 bay leaf

Salt and pepper to taste

1. Rinse the pheasant pieces and pat dry with paper towels. Put into the slow cooker. Grate off zest, and then squeeze oranges for juice. Set aside.

2. Cook pancetta in a heavy skillet over medium-high heat for about 4 minutes, or until browned. Remove from the pan with a slotted spoon, and transfer the pancetta to the slow cooker. Discard all but 2 tablespoons of the grease.

3. Add onion, carrot, celery, garlic, and sausage to the skillet. Cook, stirring frequently, for about 5 minutes, or until onion is translucent and sausage is almost cooked. Scrape mixture into the slow cooker.

4. Add tomatoes, orange zest, orange juice, stock, basil, parsley, thyme, and bay leaf to the slow cooker, and stir well. Cook on Low for 6 to 8 hours or on High for 3 to 4 hours, until vegetables are soft. Remove and discard bay leaf. Season with salt and pepper.

Pheasant is a game bird, so the meat will be leaner and tougher than that of a domestic chicken or turkey. You can often find pheasant at a farmer's market. Ask farmers you know who raise chickens and turkeys if they have pheasant or know someone who does.

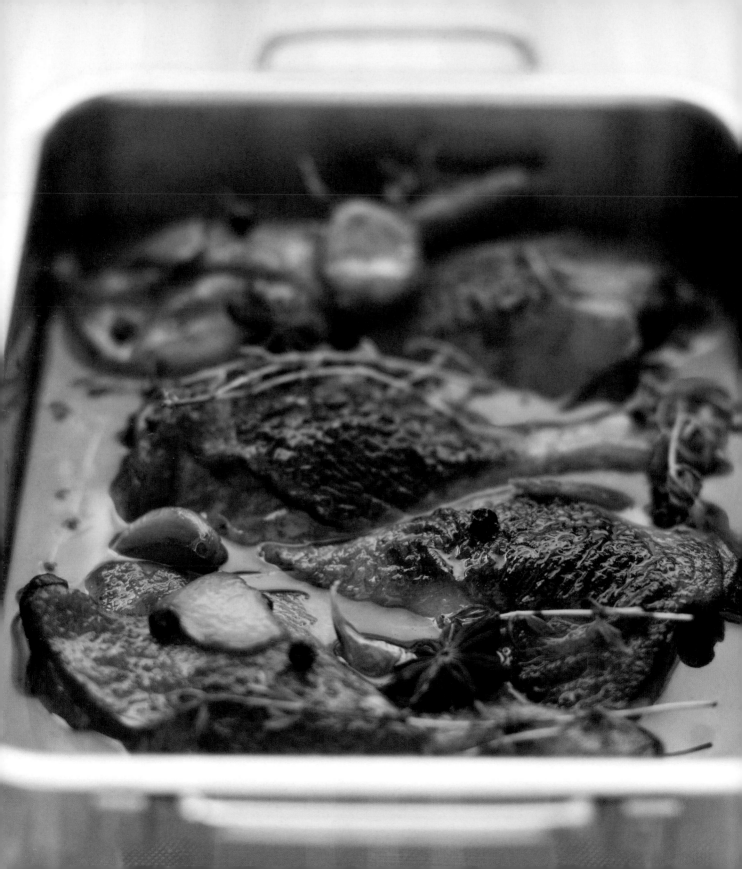

Duck Confit

In essence, this is a simple dish of cured duck legs preserved in fat. Once you taste how good this is, you'll be eager to serve your lovely confit to family and friends. You can serve it in many ways, from "as is"—the just-cooked legs themselves—to shredded over salads, over sautéed greens, or just for delicious snacking. You can use the fat for roasting winter vegetables or other meats.

Serves 6.

¼ cup kosher salt

1 tablespoon freshly ground black pepper

8 fresh thyme sprigs, leaves stripped off for use

3 bay leaves

2 teaspoons juniper berries

6 whole duck legs

2½ pounds duck fat (this will yield about 5 cups)

1. In a small bowl, combine the salt, pepper, thyme leaves, bay leaves, and juniper berries. Rinse the duck legs with cold water and pat dry with paper towels. Place in a large baking dish and spread the salt rub evenly on all sides. Cover and refrigerate overnight to cure the meat.

2. When ready to cook the legs, place the duck fat in the slow cooker and put the heat on High to melt the fat. Remove the duck legs from the refrigerator and, one at a time, take them out of the pan and rinse them under cold water. Pat them dry with paper towels. When the fat is melted, add the legs to the cooker. The fat should stay at a simmer, so you'll want to turn the heat down to Low. Cover and cook on Low for about 4 hours. When cooked, the meat will be very tender and fall away from the bones.

3. Remove the cooked legs immediately, eating them right away or allowing them to cool for later use.

4. Put the fat from the slow cooker into a glass bowl that can fit the legs back into it and that can be securely sealed. When the fat and legs have cooled, put the legs into the bowl and refrigerate. The duck confit is good this way in the fridge for about 6 months. When ready to use, just remove a leg and allow it to come to room temperature so the fat can melt before using or eating.

> Buy the duck legs and fat at a specialty butcher or grocery store, but once you have the fat, you can reuse it.

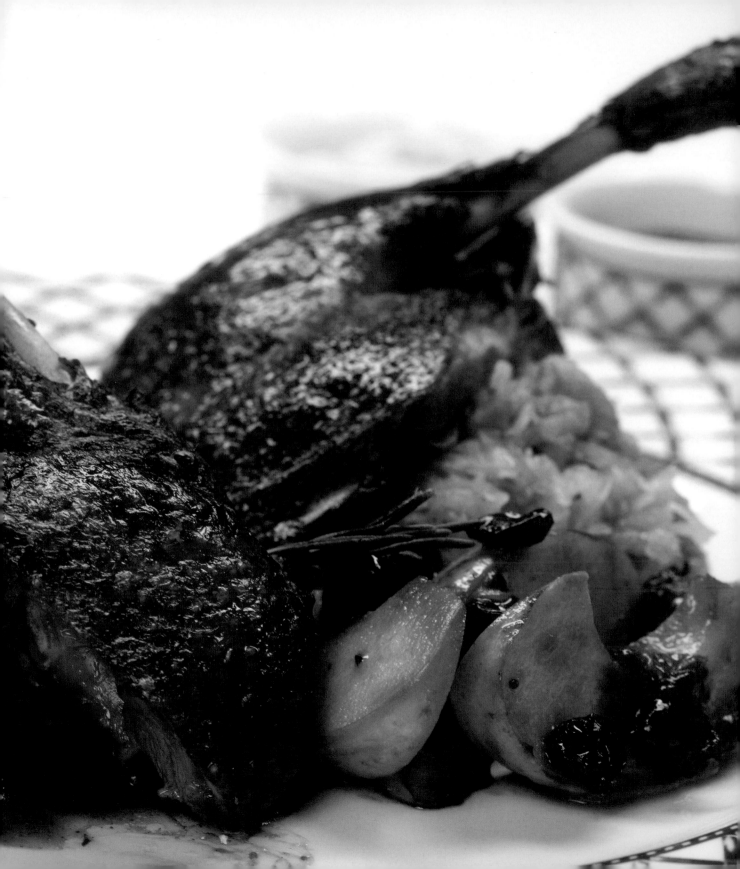

Duck with Apples and Currants

This is a fabulous fall dish since it is loaded with apples. The currants add a hint of sweetness and pair really well with the duck.

Makes 4 to 6 servings.

2 pounds fresh duck parts, skin on

8 firm, fresh baking apples, cored and cut into cubes, but not peeled

3 cloves garlic, minced

2 tablespoons dried currants

¼ teaspoon cinnamon

½ teaspoon salt

1 cup red wine

1. Rinse the duck and pat dry with paper towels. Put it in the slow cooker.

2. Add the apples, garlic, currants, cinnamon, salt, and wine, and stir to combine.

3. Cover and cook on Low for 6 to 8 hours, or on High for 4 to 5 hours, or until meat is very tender.

Variations:

* This dish can be made with pears instead of apples, or with a bit of broth.

* Turn the apple mixture into a cream sauce by adding ½ cup coconut milk into it and bringing it to a slow boil so that it blends.

Poultry Scottiglia I

The dish *Scottiglia* is essentially a stew made from whatever animals hunters could catch, cooked with whatever seasonings and vegetables were also available. The dish hails from Southern Tuscany. Because it's possible that every cook can craft a Scottiglia to their liking based on what's in their pantry, there are two recipes for Scottiglia here—and you can feel free to create others!

Makes 8 to 10 servings.

¼ cup olive oil

1 small onion, minced

1 medium carrot, peeled and minced

2 cloves garlic, pressed

½ teaspoon crushed red pepper flakes

1 pound diced boneless chicken thighs

1 pound diced boneless turkey

1 pound diced boneless duck

1 8-oz can plum tomatoes, drained and chopped

2 cups dry red wine

4 cups chicken stock

1 tablespoon fresh parsley, minced

Salt and pepper to taste

1. In a large skillet, heat 2 tablespoons of the oil and add the onion and carrot. Cook, stirring, until onions are translucent, about 3 minutes. Add the garlic and red pepper flakes, stir and cook for another minute, and transfer mix to the slow cooker.

2. Add the remaining 2 tablespoons of oil in the skillet, heat, and add the meats, stirring, until the chunks are browned on all sides. Turn off the heat and add the meat to the slow cooker.

3. Add the tomatoes, wine, chicken stock, and parsley. Cover and cook on Low for 8 to 10 hours or on High for 6 to 8 hours until the meat is very tender. Season with salt and pepper to taste.

The specific region in Southern Tuscany from which this dish hails is Maremma, which borders the Ligurian and Tyrrhenian Seas. It has a varied topography ranging from dense forests to sparkling beaches. Somewhat wild and remote, it is a place where peasant traditions have reigned for centuries, including in its cuisine.

Poultry Scottiglia II

This variation on a more classic Scottiglia features root vegetables and is more of a fall/winter dish.

Makes 8 to 10 servings.

4 tablespoons olive oil

1 medium leek, white part only, sliced thin, washed and dried

1 cup peeled and cubed butternut squash

1 medium eggplant, diced

2 cloves garlic, pressed

½ teaspoon crushed red pepper flakes

1 pound diced boneless chicken thighs

1 pound diced boneless turkey

1 pound diced boneless duck

1 8-oz can plum tomatoes, drained and chopped

2 cups dry red wine

4 cups chicken stock

1 tablespoon fresh parsley, minced

Salt and pepper to taste

1. In a large skillet, heat 2 tablespoons of the oil and add the leek and squash. Cook, stirring, until the leeks are translucent, about 3 minutes. Add the eggplant and continue to cook, stirring, for another 2 minutes until vegetables are sautéed. Add garlic and red pepper flakes, remove from heat, and transfer mix to the slow cooker.

2. Add the remaining 2 tablespoons of oil in the skillet, heat, and add the meats, stirring, until the chunks are browned on all sides.

3. Turn off the heat and add the meat to the slow cooker. Add the tomatoes, wine, chicken stock, and parsley. Cover and cook on Low for 8 to 10 hours or on High for 6 to 8 hours until the meat is very tender. Season with salt and pepper to taste.

Get your *Maremma* "flair" going and experiment with this recipe. Consider cooking with a flavored oil, like macadamia nut oil or truffle oil. Vary the types of meats used, mixing and matching with poultry and other meats. Have a Scottiglia slow cooker party and ask everyone to make their own version. Choose a wine from the area, and have a Scottiglia cookoff.

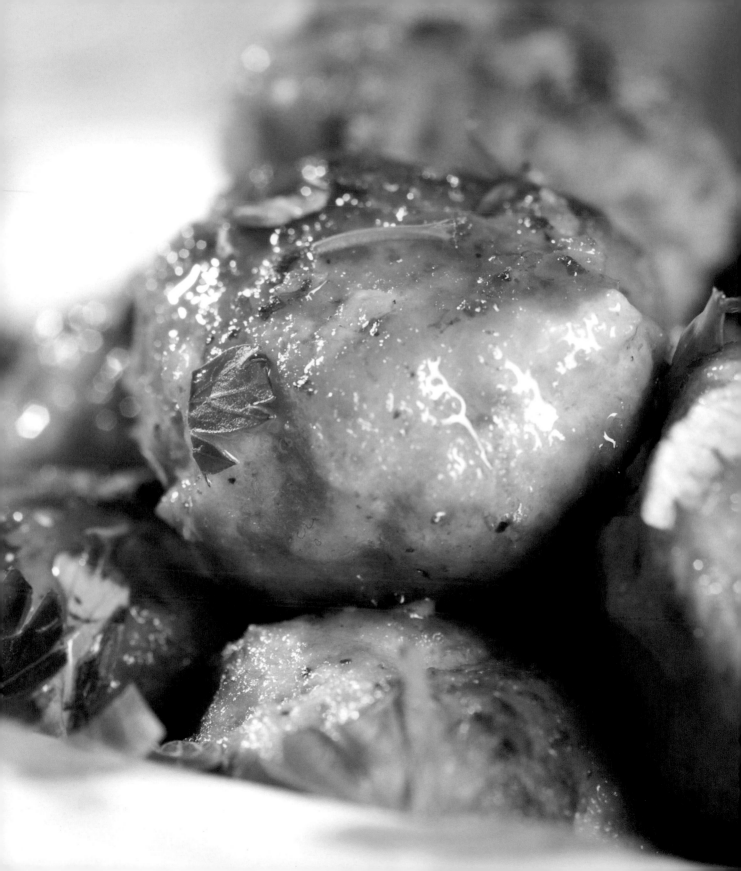

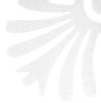

Turkey Meatballs Italiano

The special blend of herbs and spices in these meatballs gives them their Italian edge—and will keep you coming back to this recipe.

Makes about 24 small meatballs.

2 tablespoons fresh basil

2 tablespoons fresh marjoram

2 tablespoons fresh oregano

2 tablespoons fresh thyme

2 tablespoons fresh rosemary

½ onion, minced

2 pounds ground turkey

1 egg, beaten

2 tablespoons coconut oil

Salt and pepper to taste

1. Make the Italian seasoning mix by chopping the fresh herbs and combining them in a small bowl. Mix them well.

2. In a large bowl, combine the onion with the turkey and the egg. Add approximately 2 tablespoons of the herb mixture. Use a fork or your hands to combine these ingredients. Don't overmix. Form the meat mixture into meatballs and set aside on a plate.

3. In a large skillet, heat coconut oil over medium-high heat to melting. Add the meatballs (in batches, if necessary) and turn them so they turn just brown on all sides. Using a slotted spoon, transfer the browned meatballs to the slow cooker.

4. Cover and cook on Low for 3 to 4 hours, or on High for 2 to 3 hours. Sprinkle with salt and pepper before serving and additional herbs if desired.

You will have leftover chopped herbs. Put the mixture into a small bowl or bag, remove the air, and seal. Store in the refrigerator or freezer. It's great to have this herb mixture on hand. You could use it in many of the recipes in this book.

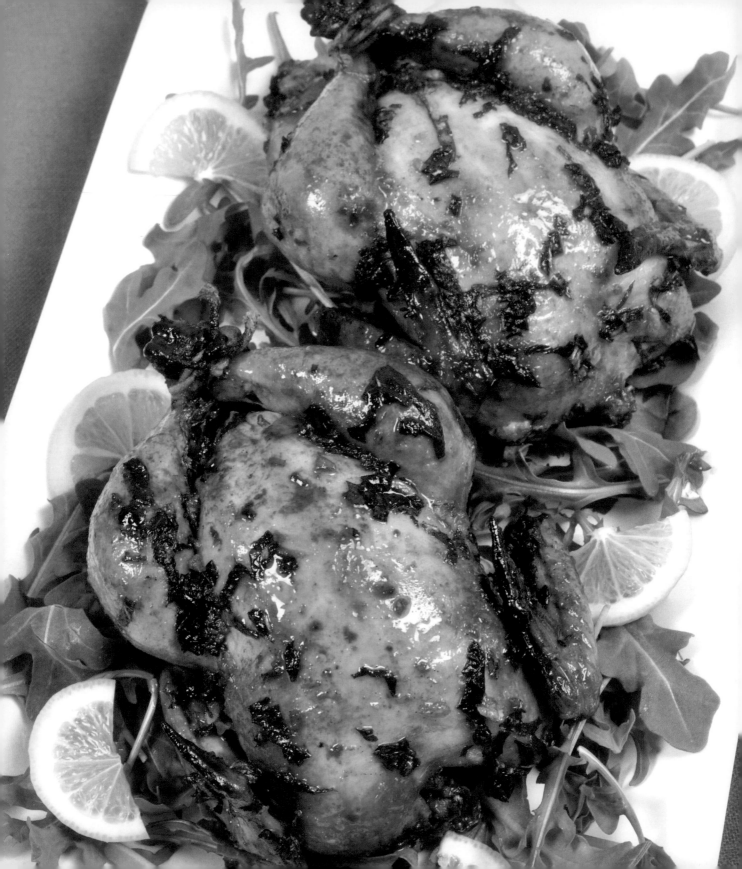

Herb-Infused Cornish Hens

Cornish hens slow-cooked with fresh herbs and lemon. Need we say more?

Makes 4 to 8 servings.

1 lemon, sliced thin

2 teaspoons olive oil

2 to 4 Cornish hens, depending on the size of your slow cooker

Salt and pepper

2 tablespoons fresh Italian seasoning mix (combination of basil, marjoram, thyme, rosemary, and oregano)

2 cloves garlic, minced fine

1. Put the lemon slices at the bottom of the slow cooker.

2. Wash and pat dry the hens. Put some olive oil on your hands and rub the outside of each hen with the oil. Place in slow cooker. Sprinkle with salt and pepper.

3. In a small bowl, combine the seasoning mix with the garlic. Sprinkle the herbs over the tops of the hens. Cover and cook on Low for 8 to 10 hours or on High for 5 to 7 hours.

4. If you want to crisp the skin when cooked through, preheat the oven to 425 degrees and when the hens are ready, transfer to a baking sheet and put in the oven for about 15 minutes.

When herbs are fresh and plentiful, buy them in bulk. They freeze beautifully and can be used separately or in combination all year.

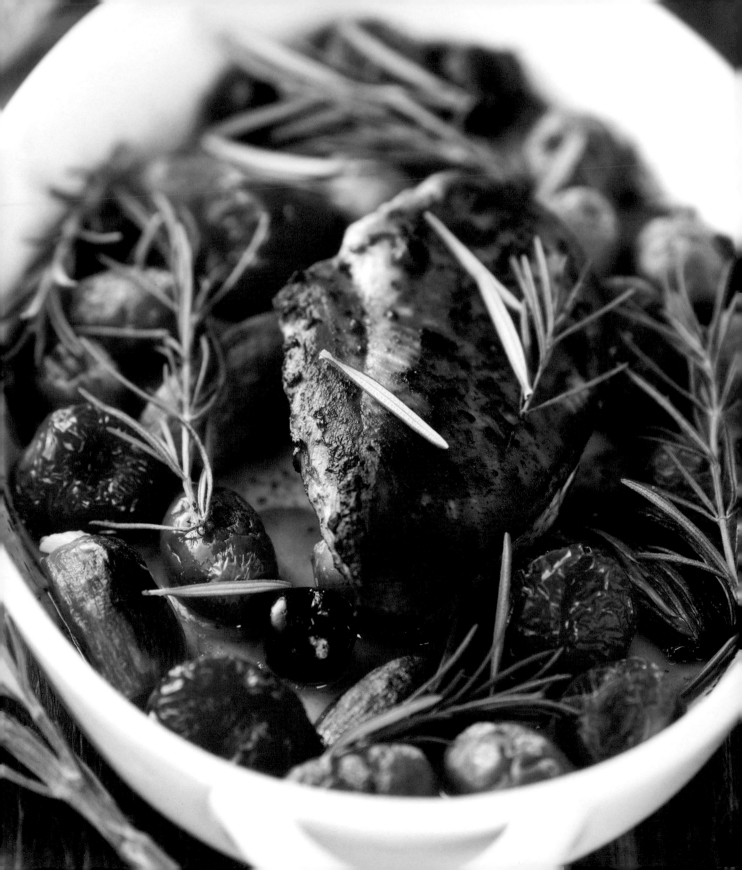

Tomato-Olive Chicken Breasts

The starts of this recipe—the tomatoes and olives—are both found throughout Italy. They make a rustic and satisfying combination that pairs especially well with tender chicken pieces.

Makes 4 to 6 servings.

3 tablespoons olive oil

1 small red or Vidalia onion, diced

5 large tomatoes, seeded and chopped into chunks

6 black olives, halved (no pits)

6 green olives, halved (no pits)

1 teaspoon capers, drained

4 boneless chicken breasts, quartered

Salt and pepper

Fresh rosemary for garnish

1. In a skillet over medium heat, add the oil and onions. Cook until the onions are translucent, about three minutes.

2. Transfer the mixture to a bowl. Add the tomatoes, olives, and capers, and stir to combine.

3. Place the slices of chicken in the slow cooker. Season with salt and pepper. Add the tomato/olive mixture on top. Cover and cook on Low for 6 to 8 hours or on High for 4 to 5 hours. Serve immediately and garnish with fresh rosemary.

> Most of us live in areas where the local supermarket has a large selection of olives, from jarred to a salad bar selection. The best olives for this recipe are fresh olives that are not from a jar and that are not kept in an oil-based sauce.

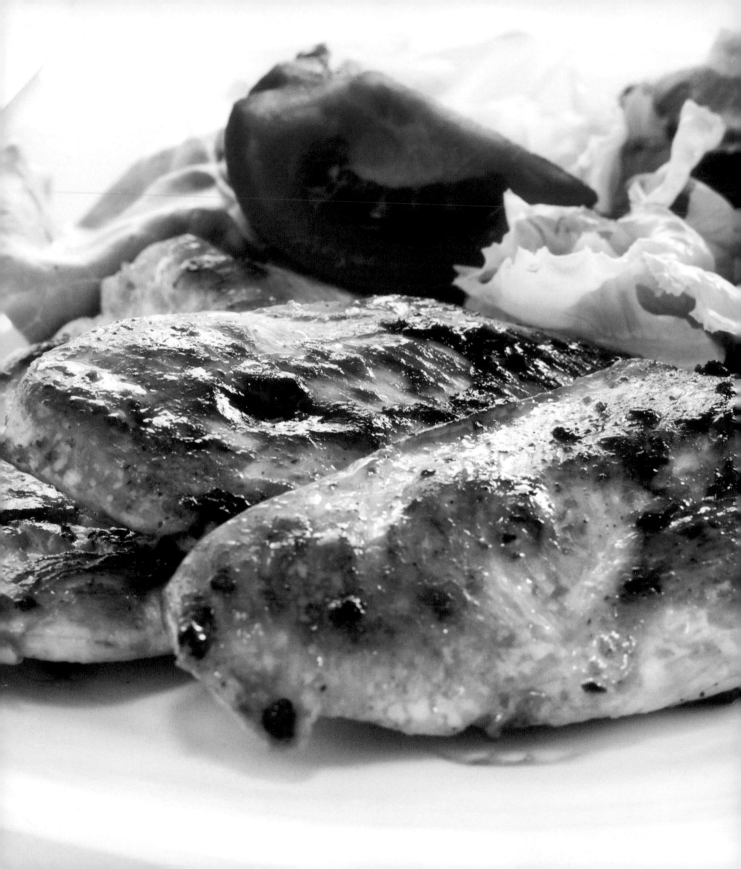

Chicken with Truffle Oil

If you're in the mood for something earthy and sublime, try this recipe. Be sure to get real truffle oil. White truffle oil from Italy is the best. It's expensive, but a little goes a long way. In fact, you'll want the smallest bottle available.

Makes 6 to 8 servings.

2 large onions, thickly sliced

2 medium carrots, peeled and cut into sticks

2 ribs celery, ends trimmed and cut into sticks

1 bay leaf

3 pounds chicken pieces, bone in, skins removed

2 tablespoons olive oil

Salt and pepper

½ teaspoon dried thyme

½ teaspoon dried sage

White truffle oil

1. In a large bowl, combine the onions, carrot sticks, and celery sticks. Place the vegetables at the bottom of the slow cooker. Add the bay leaf.

2. When skins are removed from the chicken pieces, wash and dry them. Put the olive oil on your hands and rub the pieces, then place them in the slow cooker. Season with the salt, pepper, thyme, and sage. Cover and cook on Low for 10 to 12 hours or on High for 5 to 7 hours.

3. Transfer chicken pieces to a serving dish. Scoop out the vegetables and place around the chicken. Drizzle with the truffle oil and serve.

> Truffles are a type of fungus, like mushrooms, but they grow underground. They have synergistic relationships with the trees that grow near them. For example, Italian white truffles are found most often in wooded areas where oak, hazel, poplar, and beech trees predominate. This is most commonly in the northern Piedmont area. Truffles are hunted with specially trained dogs or pigs.

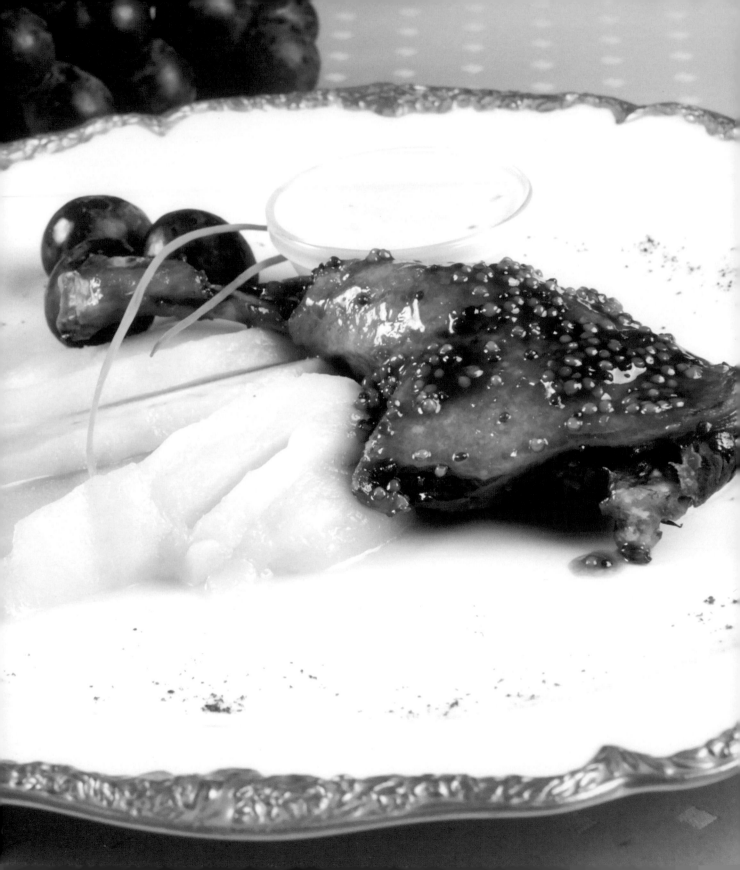

Duck on a Bed of Pears

Pears grown in cooler climates ripen in late summer/early fall. They are a fruit with a strong association with the end-of-year holidays. This recipe is an elegant one to serve for company at that time of year.

Makes 4 to 6 servings.

4-pound duck, cut into pieces

3 leeks

3 tablespoons ghee

½ cup water

8 pears, not quite ripe

¼ cup dried cranberries (not sweetened)

Salt and pepper to taste

1. Cut the duck into large pieces, working with the bones. Keep the skin on the duck. Wash and pat dry the pieces. Set aside.

2. Cut the rooted bottom off the leeks. Work with the whitest part of the leeks, cutting off the green top. Slice the leeks into ¼-inch rounds, and rinse them in a colander as many times as necessary to remove any sand that may be there.

3. Heat the ghee in a skillet over medium heat and add the leeks, stirring and cooking until translucent, about 3 minutes. Transfer to the slow cooker.

4. Cut the top off and core the pears, and cut them into cubes. Put the pears on top of the leek mixture. Add the duck pieces, and season with salt and pepper. Cover and cook on Low for 10 to 12 hours or on High for 6 to 8 hours until the duck is very tender.

5. Transfer the duck to a platter and cover with foil to keep warm. Add the cranberries to the leek and pear mixture, and continue to cook on Low for about 20 minutes. Serve the leeks on the side.

Duck meat is loaded with iron—more per serving than chicken, turkey, and even certain cuts of beef. Iron is essential for a healthy immune system, as it supports red blood cells that transport nutrients in the body. When cooked, the meat is red, just like a lean cut of beef.

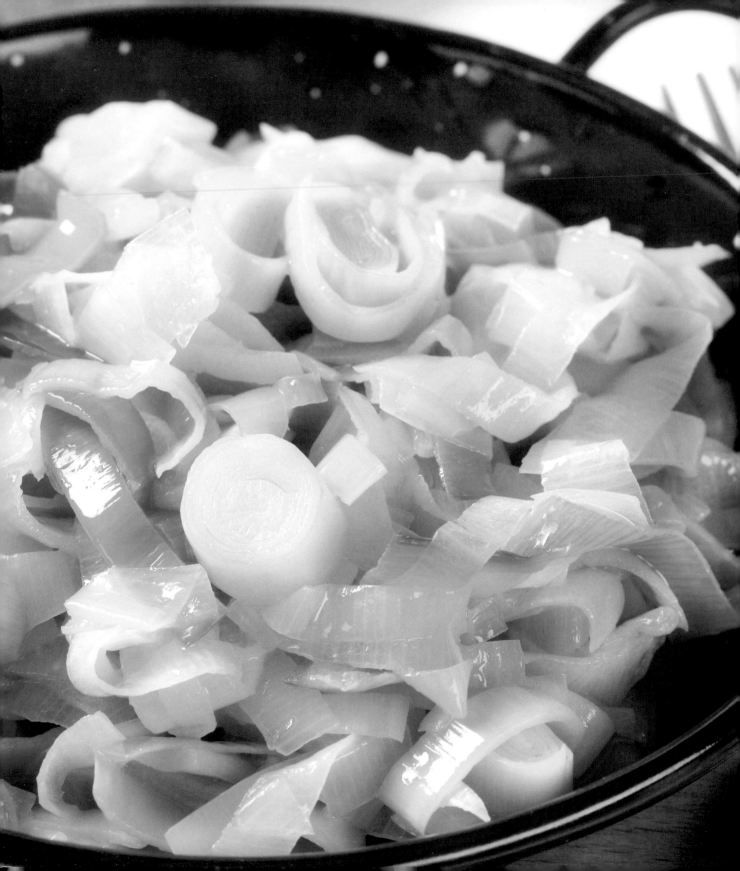

Chicken with Leeks and Walnut Oil

Slow cooking chicken with leeks almost guarantees a delicious meal because of the way the leeks moisten and soften in the chicken juices. Drizzling walnut oil over this dish takes it to a whole other level.

Makes 4 to 6 servings.

4 leeks

1 tablespoon ghee or olive oil

3 ribs celery, leafy top and tough bottom discarded, then diced

3 cloves garlic, crushed

Pinch of cayenne pepper

1 cup chicken stock

3 pounds skinless, bone-in chicken thighs

Salt and pepper

¼ cup walnut oil

½ cup chopped fresh parsley

1. Prepare leeks by cutting the rooted bottoms off them and cutting away the part where the leeks turn greener so that you're using the whitest part of the plant. Slice the leeks into ¼-inch rounds, and rinse them in a colander as many times as necessary to remove any sand that might be there.

2. In a skillet, heat the ghee or oil and add the leeks, celery, and garlic. Cook, stirring, for about 3 minutes or until the leeks are translucent. Add the pinch of cayenne and mix.

3. Transfer the leek mixture to the slow cooker and add the chicken stock. Place the thighs in the slow cooker and sprinkle with salt and pepper. Cover and cook on Low for 6 to 8 hours or on High for 4 to 6 hours. Transfer the meat and leeks to a platter. Combine the walnut oil and parsley, stir to combine, and sprinkle/drizzle over the meat.

Walnuts are a prized ingredient in Italian home cooking. They are harvested in the fall and stored for use throughout the winter and the following year. Walnuts have some outstanding nutritional benefits. Besides being high in omega-3 fatty acids, they have been proven to lower cholesterol levels and reduce the risk of heart disease.

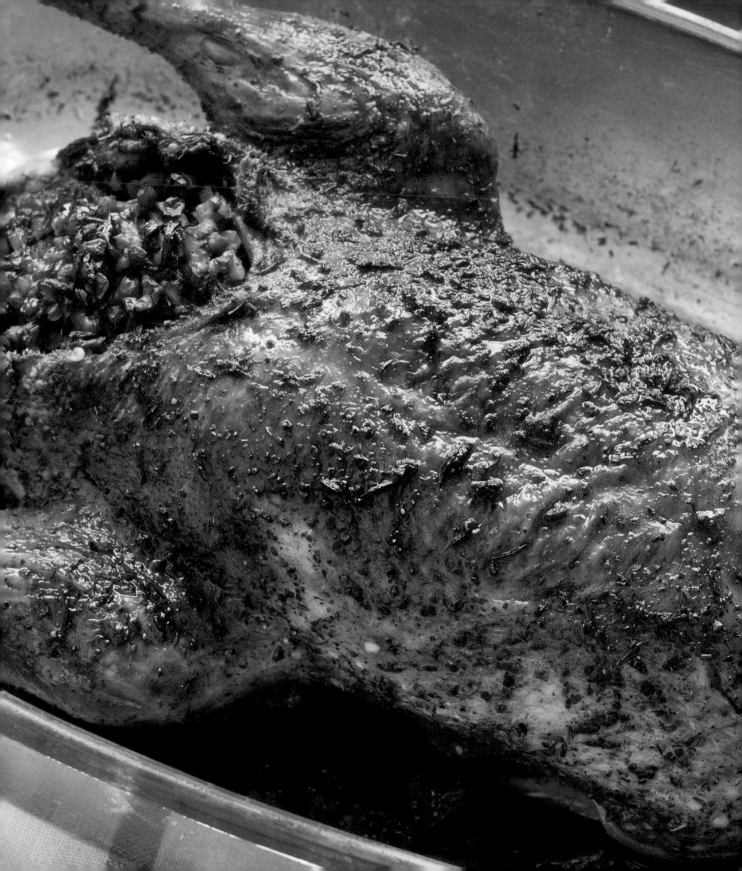

Arnata alla Novarese (Duck Novarese)

For a really festive and fun occasion, take a shot at this decadent Italian concoction—a duck stuffed with meat and vegetables! It takes some preparation, but the result is fabulous!

Makes 6 to 8 servings.

1 small head cauliflower

3 tablespoons coconut oil

1 tablespoon fresh parsley, chopped

Salt and pepper

2 eggs

1 onion, chopped

4 oz. pancetta, diced

½ pound ground veal

½ pound sweet Italian sausage, casing removed

2 carrots, chopped

1 stalk celery, chopped

2 cloves garlic, minced

4- to 5 pound duck

1 cup chicken stock

1. Remove any leaves from the cauliflower and cut out the bottom stalk. Break apart into florets. Process the florets in a food processor or in batches, forming rice-sized pieces. Transfer the chopped cauliflower to a bowl. When all is processed, heat 1 tablespoon of the coconut oil in a skillet and add the cauliflower. Cook, stirring, until cauliflower is al dente, about 6 to 8 minutes. Transfer the cooked cauliflower back into the bowl and stir in the parsley. Season with salt and pepper.

2. Put the remaining 2 tablespoons of the oil in the skillet and heat. Add the onion and pancetta and cook, stirring, until onion softens, about 3 minutes. Add the veal and sausage and continue to cook and stir for another 3 minutes. Add the carrot, celery, and garlic and stir to combine thoroughly. Transfer meat mixture to a large bowl. Add the eggs and cauliflower and combine thoroughly with the other ingredients.

3. Stuff the duck with the mixture, securing the cavity by tying the legs together with kitchen string. Place the duck in the slow cooker. Add the chicken stock. Cover and cook on Low for 10 to 12 hours or on High for 6 to 8 hours, or until duck is tender and juices flow clear from cavity. Transfer to a platter and serve.

Novarese refers to the style of the dish, which originated in Novara, Italy. Novara is in the Piedmont region of the country, in the northwest. The use of several meats in this recipe—like the one for Scottiglia—reflects the practicality of the cuisine. It combines the flavors and textures of what is available in the area. The classic recipe calls for rice; this Paleo version uses cauliflower "rice" as a substitute.

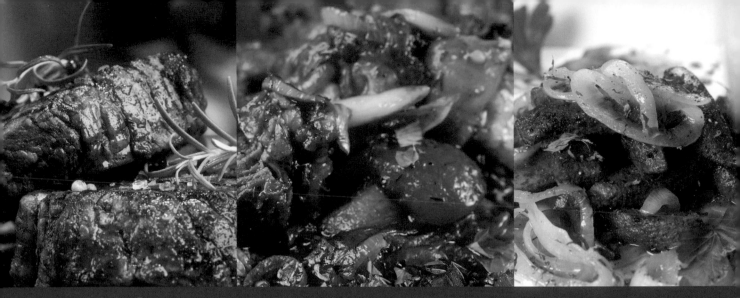

Chapter 6

Paleo *Secondi:*

Beef, Pork, Lamb, and Game

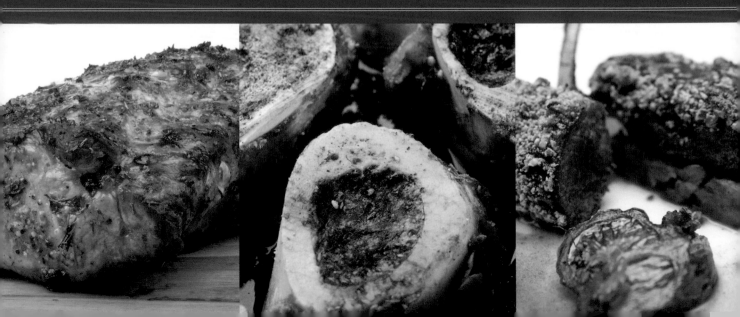

This chapter showcases recipes featuring traditional and classic Italian meat combinations, like sausage and peppers, roast young lamb, and hearty veal stew. It also features some recipes that our Italian ancestors might have been more comfortable and familiar with than we are but that are equally worth trying: dishes like roast heart, pigs' feet, and sweetbreads. Welcome to the magic of slow cooking, where, with the right ingredients, nearly anything can be made tender and delicious. This is true of the organs and other odd cuts that find their way into this chapter. I keep coming back to the words of the late, great Marcella Hazan, who said that taste is everything. Things don't have to be complicated to taste good. Work with good ingredients and you're on the right track. And remember, again, that it's about sharing food and bringing people together.

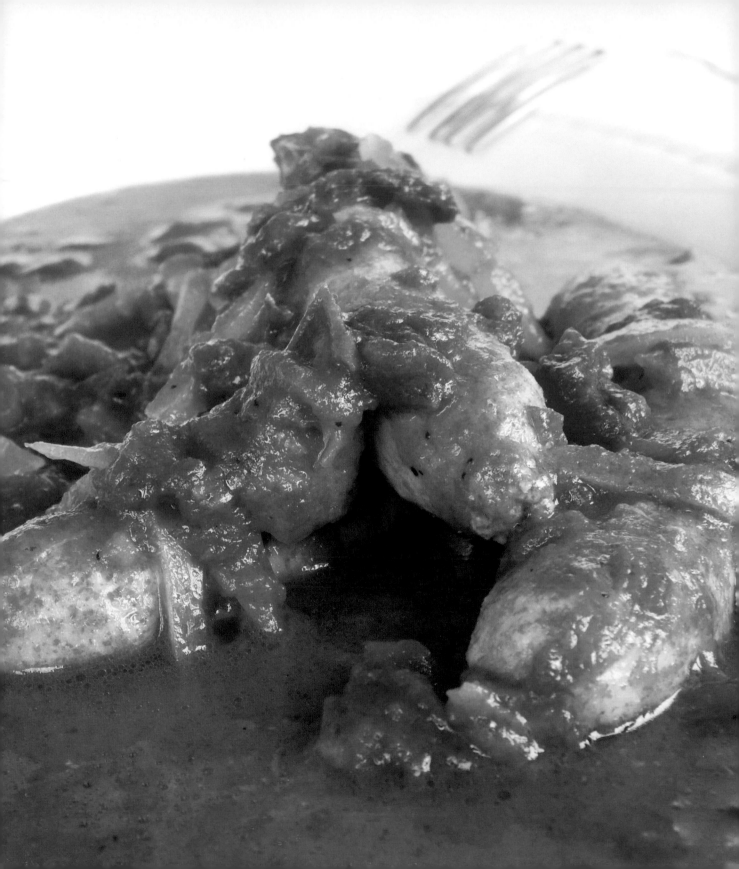

Sausage and Pepper Stew

Anyone who shares meals with Italians knows that this is a classic combo of ingredients and flavors. This thick stew is wonderful accompanied by a salad of fresh greens.

Makes 6 to 8 servings.

1 pound sweet Italian sausage

1 pound hot Italian sausage

1 tablespoon clarified butter

1 onion, thinly sliced

2 bell peppers, seeded and chopped

3 cloves garlic, minced

1 14.5-oz can stewed tomatoes

2 cups chicken stock or broth

1 teaspoon fresh oregano, chopped (or ½ teaspoon dried)

1 teaspoon fresh thyme, chopped (or ½ teaspoon dried)

Salt and pepper to taste

1. Cut the sausages into ¼-inch slices. In a large skillet over medium-high heat, cook the sausages, turning frequently, until browned on both sides. Work in batches if all the meat doesn't fit easily.

2. Remove the browned sausage with a slotted spoon and put it in the slow cooker.

3. Add the clarified butter and the onions to the skillet, and sauté for a couple of minutes until just translucent. Add the peppers and garlic, and cook for another 3 to 5 minutes.

4. Scrape the onion-pepper-garlic mixture into the slow cooker. Top with the tomatoes and broth, and sprinkle the herbs on top. Cover and cook on Low for 5 to 6 hours or on High for 2 to 3 hours. Season with salt and pepper.

Variations:

* If you want a spicier dish, use only hot sausage; if you prefer a milder dish, use only sweet sausage.
* You can also increase the color by using different colored peppers— a combo of green, red, and even orange if you'd like.

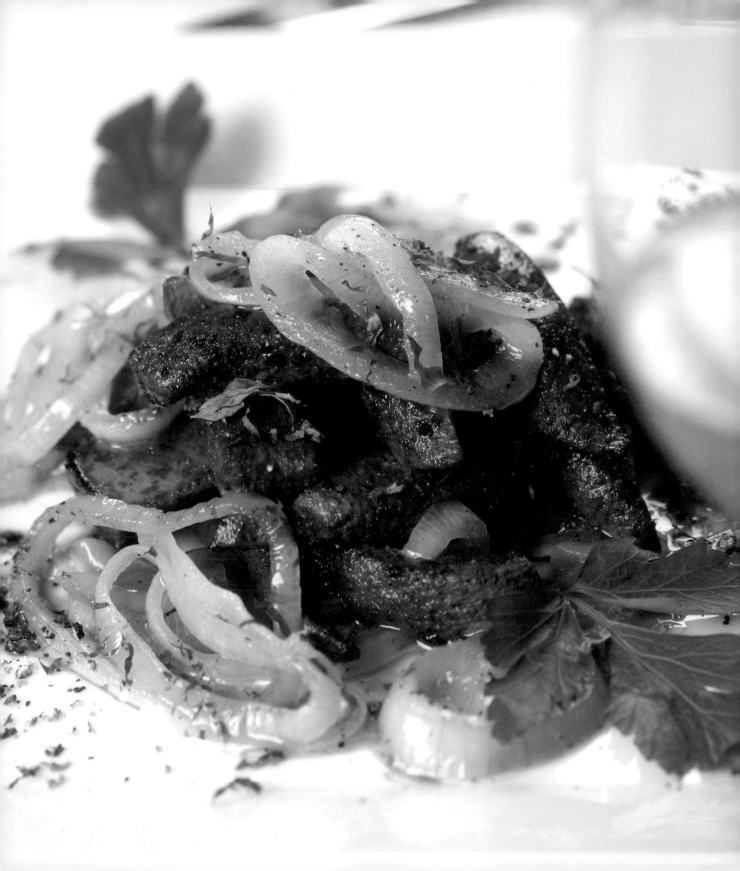

Liver and Onions

If you're a liver skeptic, try this recipe and see if it changes your mind. The slow cooker is magic for offal—*not awful!*— meats like this.

Makes 2 to 4 servings.

6 slices bacon

2 pounds calf or beef liver

6 yellow onions, peeled and sliced into ¼-inch wedges

1 cup water

Salt and pepper to taste

1 tablespoon fresh parsley, chopped

1. Cook the bacon in a skillet on medium-high heat, transferring it to a plate covered with paper towels when cooked crisp. In the skillet with the bacon fat, fry the liver to lightly brown it on both sides—about 2 minutes a side.

2. Put the liver in the slow cooker and cover with the onions. Crumble and add the bacon, then top with the water. Cover and cook on Low for 6 to 8 hours. Don't cook this on High.

3. Season with salt and pepper to taste, and garnish with parsley when serving.

> **Liver is actually a super-food, loaded with protein, vitamins, and minerals and low in fat. While it is high in cholesterol, its benefits outweigh that one shortcoming, and it's truthfully not eaten frequently enough for that to matter for most people. In some cultures, the liver of fresh-killed game is the "prize" for the hunter who makes the kill, and it is eaten fresh out of the animal as it is butchered. Slow-cooking with delicious onions and smoky bacon is more to our liking.**

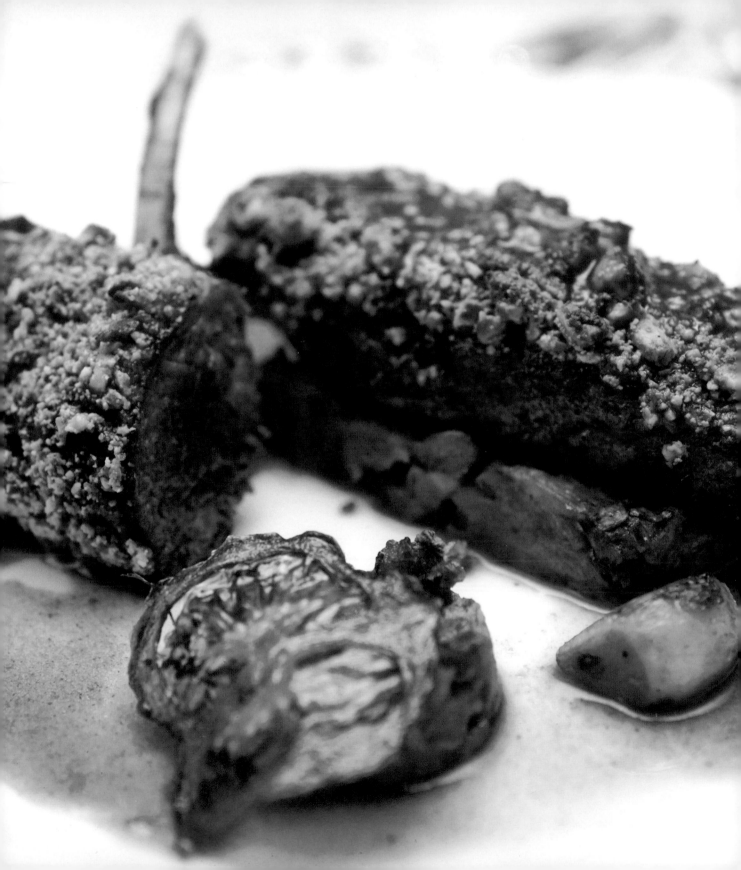

Pistachio-Crusted Lamb

If you want crunchy pistachios and lamb on the rare side, cook the chops under the broiler. But if you want flavors that slow-cook together for a juicy finish, make it in the slow cooker.

Makes 2 to 4 servings.

1 cup unsalted shelled pistachios, finely chopped

2 tablespoons honey

1 tablespoon fresh lemon juice

1 teaspoon ground cumin

¼ teaspoon cayenne

1½ pounds lamb rib chops

2 tablespoons olive oil

Salt and pepper to taste

1. Put the finely chopped pistachios in a wide-brimmed soup dish. In another dish like this, mix the honey and lemon juice, and in a third, combine the cumin and cayenne. The chops will be dipped in all of these on their way to the slow cooker.

2. Brush the chops with the olive oil, dip and flip in the cumin/cayenne blend, and season with some salt and pepper. In a skillet over medium-high heat, brown the chops on both sides, about 5 minutes a side. When browned, dip both sides of the chop in the honey/lemon combo, and then in the pistachios.

3. Position the chops in the slow cooker. Cook on Low for about 3 hours or on High for about 2 hours so the meat isn't overdone.

Pistachios are grown on tall bushes and originated in the Middle East. Today, Iran, Turkey, and the United States are the three biggest growers of pistachios. They need a particular kind of soil and climate. In Italy, they are grown in Sicily, where they are a prized treat. Most often you find pistachio as a flavor of gelato. This recipe shows off a zestier pistachio flavor.

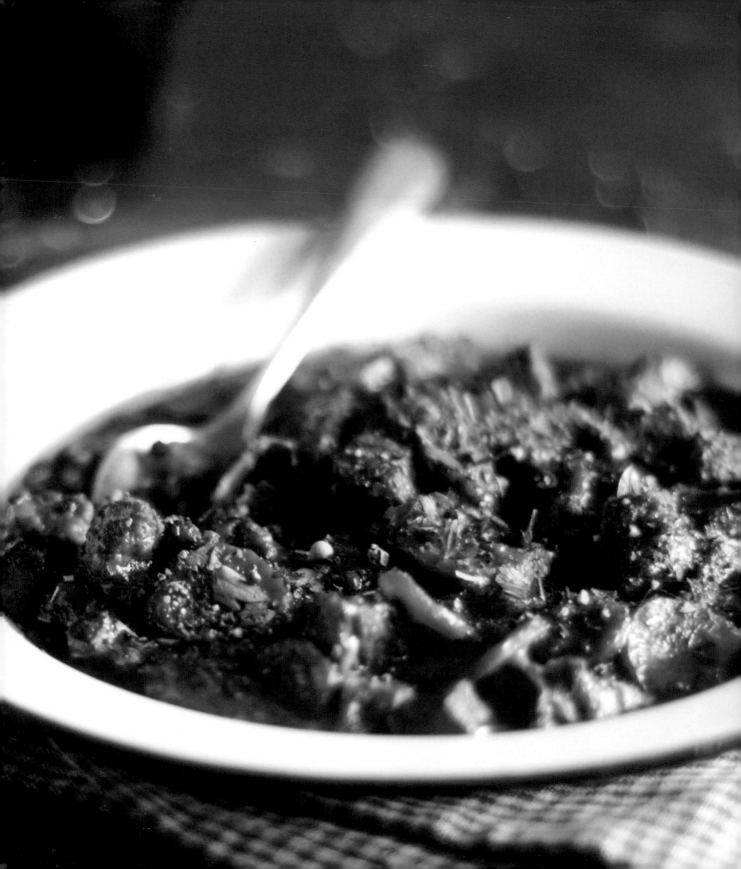

Venison Stew

This is the kind of rich and delicious meal you want to make for a long winter's night.

Makes 6 to 8 servings.

1 4-pound venison shoulder

Salt and pepper to taste

4 to 6 slices bacon

¼ cup bacon drippings

2 onions, diced

1 carrot, peeled and diced

1 stalk celery, diced

¼ cup almond flour

1 12-oz can diced tomatoes

½ cup mushrooms, sliced

2 cloves garlic, crushed

3 cups beef stock or broth

1 cup red wine

1 sprig fresh thyme

1 sprig fresh rosemary

2 bay leaves

1. Season the venison with salt and pepper. In a heavy-bottomed skillet, cook the bacon, reserving the cooked strips. In the bacon drippings, cook the venison so that it is browned on all sides. Put the venison in the slow cooker.

2. Into the skillet, add the onions, carrots, and celery, and stir frequently until they have browned slightly. Add the almond flour and stir to combine. Put the mixture into the slow cooker with the venison.

3. In a large bowl, combine the tomatoes, mushrooms, garlic, beef stock, red wine, thyme, rosemary, and bay leaves. Pour this over and around the venison. Cook on Low for 6 to 8 hours or on High for 5 to 7 hours.

Eating venison (the meat of deer, but also antelope, elk, and reindeer) and other game meats is a true Paleo experience—though we're lucky to have the herbs and spices we are used to seasoning it with. Venison is rich in B vitamins, iron, and phosphorous but low in fat and cholesterol.

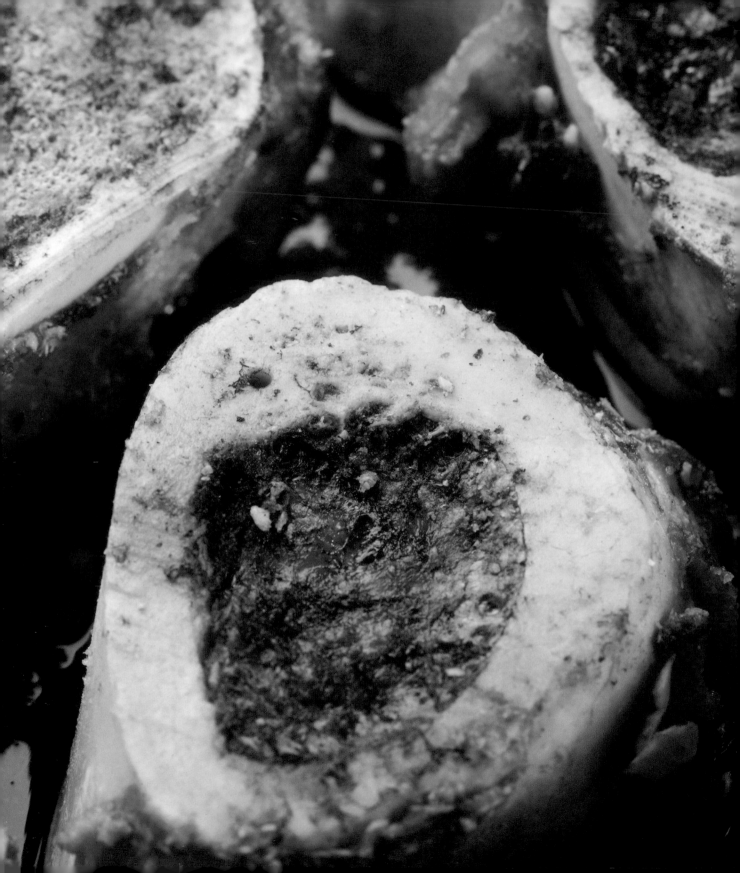

Magical Marrow Bones

Our Paleo ancestors would be sure to eat all the marrow from the bones of the animals they killed for food, and we should, too. Here is a recipe for easy beef marrow bones.

Serves 4 to 6.

3 or 4 large beef bones with lots of marrow
Salt and pepper to taste

1. Prep the bones for cooking by soaking to remove the blood. Place the bones in a large bowl of ice water, adding a teaspoon of salt for every cup of water. Put the bowl in the refrigerator, and change the salt water every 6 hours. Do this for 12 to 24 hours, and be sure to either use the bones within 24 hours of completing this, or freeze them immediately (for up to 3 months).

2. Put the bones in the slow cooker so the part that you would scoop the marrow out from is facing up. Cook on Low for about 2 hours or on High for about 1 hour.

3. When the marrow is melting and hot, it's ready. Scoop it out of the bones and enjoy it right then and there, with a sprinkle of salt and freshly ground black pepper.

Bone marrow is fat, but it's a monounsaturated fat, so it's all good fat. It is also rich in protein, iron, and calcium. While it is rare to find someone 50 years old or younger in the United States who has eaten bone marrow, it is not uncommon for older people, particularly of European descent, to have had it. If you're a fan of the crisp, fatty part of foods like bacon, ribs, and chops, you should enjoy these very much. Be sure to purchase them from a farmer of grass-fed beef and ask them to cut them for you.

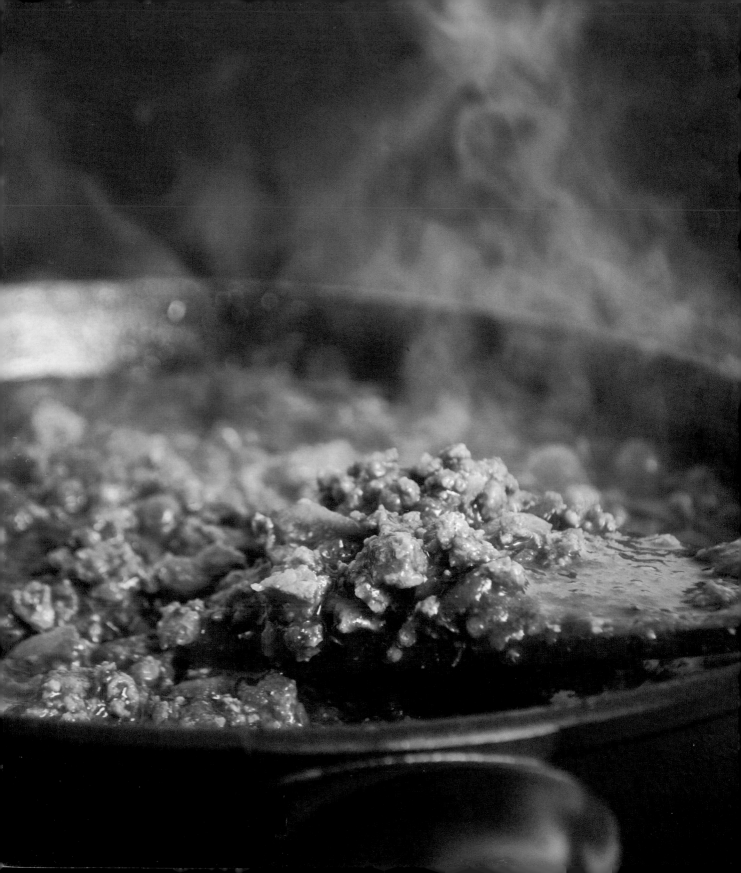

Ragu Italiano (Spaghetti Sauce)

The Bolognese, who have a style of sauce named after them that's considered the very best, call their sauce a ragu, which is a thick, rich sauce. This is the ultimate Italian food, one that sons for centuries have been measuring their future wives by—if she can make this as good as his mother, she's a keeper.

Makes 4 to 8 servings.

2 tablespoons olive oil

2 carrots, sliced

Pepper

1 onion, chopped fine

2 stalks celery, chopped

8 oz button mushrooms, rinsed and sliced thick

1 pound ground beef

1 pound ground veal

2 14.5-oz cans diced tomatoes, undrained

3 cloves garlic, minced

2 teaspoons dried oregano

1 tablespoon dried basil

1 teaspoon red pepper flakes

Salt and pepper to taste

1. In a large skillet over medium-high heat, add the olive oil, carrots, pepper, onion, celery, and mushrooms. Cook, stirring, for about 3 minutes, and put in the bottom of the slow cooker.

2. In the same skillet, brown the ground meats together over medium heat, being careful not to cook too long. The meat should be slightly pink. Put it in the slow cooker on top of the vegetables.

3. Add the tomatoes, garlic, oregano, basil, and red pepper flakes. Stir to combine.

4. Cover and cook on Low for 5 to 7 hours or on High for about 3 hours. Season with salt and pepper.

While you can't eat pasta on the Paleo diet, you can make a delightful bowl of spaghetti squash upon which to serve this sauce. You can also slice long zucchini with a mandoline to make "noodles," steam the ribbons, and serve the ragu atop the zucchini noodles.

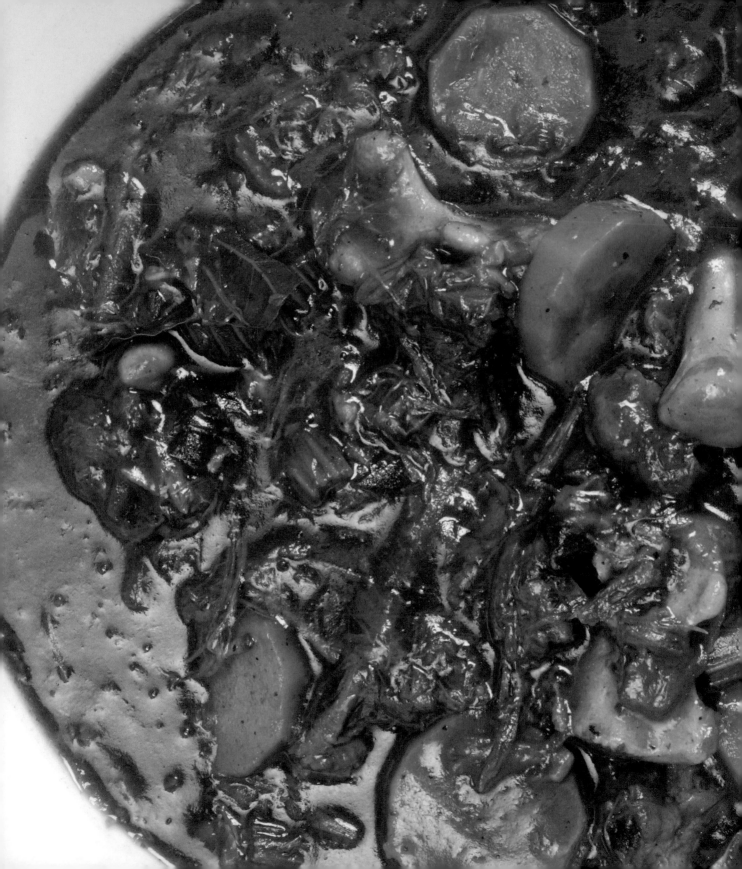

Oxtail Stew

This is another powerhouse of a Paleo meal, full of the rich goodness of fatty meat and fall vegetables. Start it the day before you're planning to serve it, as you'll need time to separate some of the cooked fat from the dish.

Makes 4 to 6 servings.

2 to 3 pounds beef oxtail

½ cup almond flour

Salt and pepper

3 tablespoons olive oil

1 cup carrots, sliced

1 cup leeks, white part only, sliced thin

4 cloves garlic, minced

½ cup mushrooms, sliced

½ cup parsnips, peeled and cubed

1 cup red wine

2 cups chicken or vegetable stock or broth

2 bay leaves

1 sprig thyme

¼ teaspoon sage

Fresh parsley, chopped, for garnish

1. Put the oxtail pieces in a large bowl, and sprinkle the almond flour, salt, and pepper over them. Turn and shake the pieces to cover with flour.

2. Heat the oil in a large, heavy bottomed skillet. Remove the oxtail pieces from the flour one by one, shaking to remove excess flour, and put them in the skillet so that all sides are browned. As they're finished, transfer the oxtails to the slow cooker. Remove pan from heat.

3. Add carrots, leeks, garlic, mushrooms, parsnips, red wine, stock, bay leaves, thyme, and sage to the slow cooker. Cover and cook on Low for 8 to 10 hours or on High for about 6 hours, finishing with an hour at Low. After cooking time, turn the slow cooker off and allow everything to cool. There will be a lot of fat in the liquid. With a slotted spoon, transfer the solids to a large serving dish. Cover and refrigerate.

4. Pour the liquid into a bowl and refrigerate it for several hours or overnight, until the fat solidifies. Scoop it out and discard it.

5. The slow-cooked meat and vegetables will be quite soft when you go to reheat them. If desired, add additional vegetables that are just cooked—carrots, green beans, or leafy greens like kale or spinach—and stir them in as the meat is reheating. Heat the stock separately and serve as gravy on the side. Garnish with fresh parsley.

> **Oxtail is literally the tail of the ox—or cow. When the animal is butchered, the tail is cut off and skinned, and the bony, muscular tail is cut into segments. It is considered "offal," like other odd parts, and is prepared different ways in different culture. It is an excellent bone from which to make stock, too.**

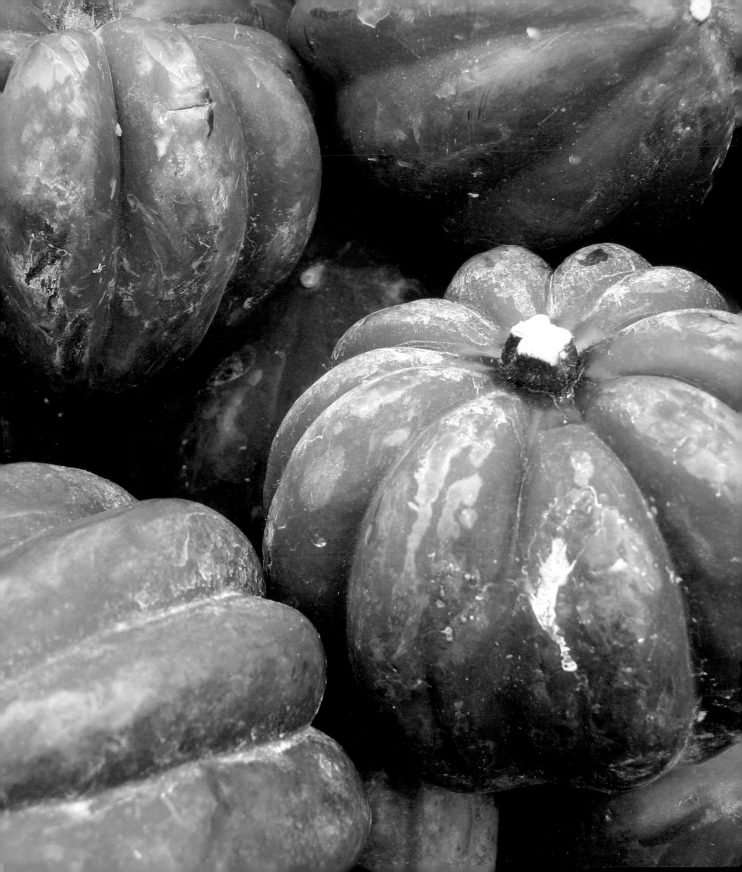

Stew with Acorn Squash

For this tasty stew, you can use beef or veal—or even cuts of game meat. The acorn squash gives a great color and flavor.

Makes 4 to 6 servings.

½ cup almond flour

2 pounds stew meat, beef or veal, fat trimmed, cut into 1-inch cubes

¼ cup olive oil

1 onion, diced

2 cloves garlic, minced

1 cup red wine

½ cup chicken stock or broth

1-pound acorn squash, peeled, seeded, and cut into cubes

2 tablespoons fresh parsley, chopped

2 teaspoons fresh thyme

Salt and pepper to taste

1. Put flour in a large bowl and add meat, stirring to coat.

2. Heat oil in a large skillet and add meat pieces, shaking off excess flour as you transfer them from the bowl to the skillet. Brown the meat on all sides. Use a slotted spoon to put browned pieces in the slow cooker.

3. Add onion and garlic to the skillet and cook, stirring, for about 3 minutes. Scrape this onto the meat in the slow cooker.

4. Add wine and stock to the skillet and bring to a boil, dislodging the browned bits in the pan. Pour mixture into the slow cooker. Add squash, parsley, and thyme to the slow cooker, and stir well.

5. Cook on Low for 6 to 8 hours or on High for 3 to 4 hours, or until meat is tender. Season to taste with salt and pepper.

Along with tomatoes and potatoes, squash is a recent addition to European cuisines and came from the New World. Squash seeds have been found in ancient Mexican archaeological digs dating back to somewhere between 9000 and 4000 BCE. The first European settlers originally thought squash to be a type of melon since they had never seen them before.

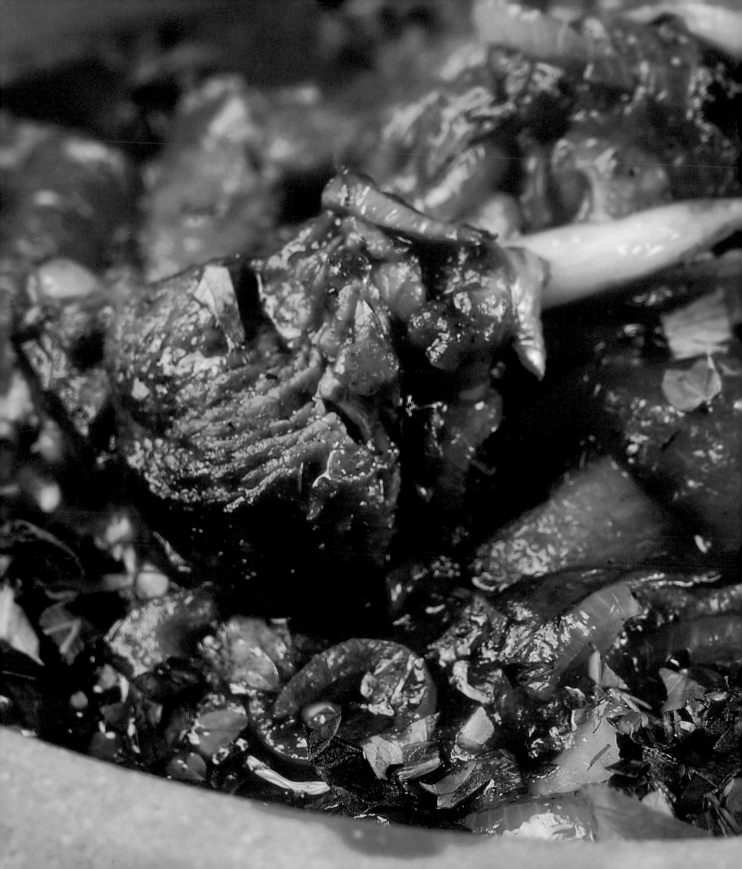

Lamb Stew with Prosciutto and Bell Peppers

Lamb is an inherently rich meat, and the sweetness of red bell peppers combined with bits of salty prosciutto serve as perfect foils to that richness.

Makes 4 to 6 servings.

2 pounds boneless lamb shoulder or leg of lamb, fat trimmed and cut into cubes

½ cup almond flour

¼ cup olive oil

1 onion, diced

3 cloves garlic, minced

¼ pound prosciutto, cut into ½-inch chunks

1 cup dry red wine

1 cup beef stock or broth

2 tablespoons fresh sage, chopped

2 tablespoons fresh parsley, chopped

2 tablespoons fresh rosemary, chopped

1 large red bell pepper, seeds and ribs removed, thinly sliced

Salt and pepper to taste

1. Put flour in a large bowl and add meat, stirring to coat.

2. Heat oil in a large skillet and add meat pieces, shaking off excess flour as you transfer them from the bowl to the skillet. Brown the meat on all sides. Use a slotted spoon to put browned pieces in the slow cooker.

3. Add prosciutto, onion, and garlic to the skillet and cook, stirring, for about 3 minutes. Scrape this onto the meat in the slow cooker.

4. Add onion and garlic to the skillet and cook, stirring, for about 3 minutes. Scrape this onto the meat in the slow cooker.

5. Add wine to the skillet, and bring to a boil, stirring to dislodge the brown bits in the skillet. Pour mixture into the slow cooker. Add stock, sage, parsley, and rosemary to the slow cooker, and stir well. Cook on Low for 6 to 8 hours or on High for 3 to 4 hours, or until lamb is almost tender. If cooking on low, raise heat to high. Add peppers, and cook for about an hour longer, or until lamb is tender. Season with salt and pepper.

> This recipe calls for meat cut away from the bones, but by all means save those bones! Add them to your next batch of beef stock to make something with a bit more earthiness and depth.

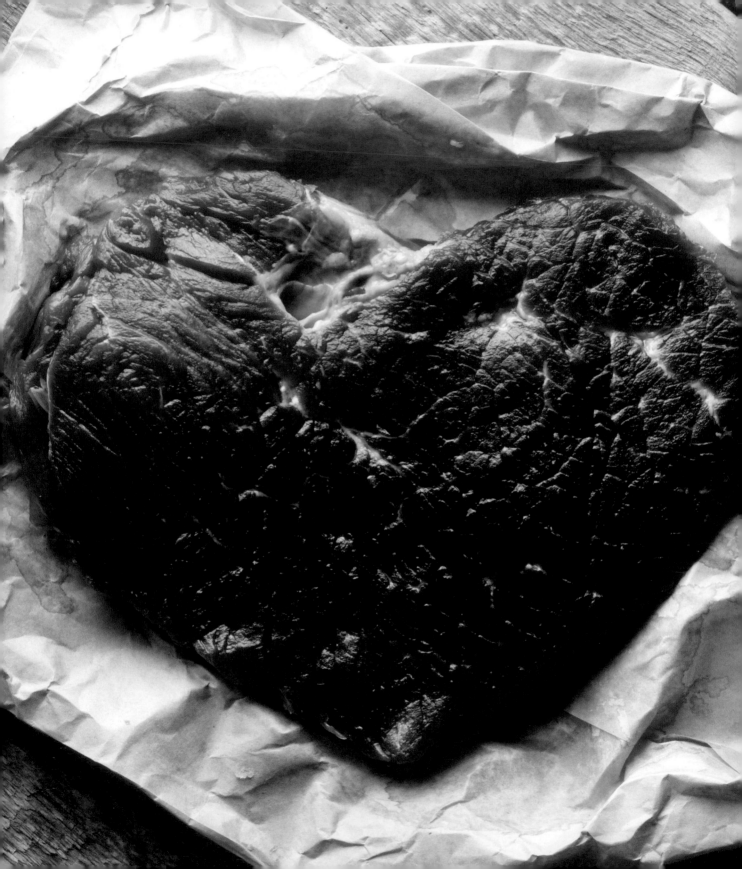

Simple but Satisfying Heart

Paleo people tend to have great relationships with local farmers and butchers. These are the folks who will turn you on to great cuts of organ meats like beef heart. Heart is a muscle like other cuts of beef, and the flavor is similar—but there's even more protein in it, along with other minerals, vitamins and even skin- and joint-enhancing amino acids. So don't let this great piece of the animal get by you.

Makes 6 to 8 servings.

1 3-4 lb beef heart

2 tablespoons olive oil

1 tablespoon balsamic vinegar

3 cloves garlic, pressed

1 teaspoon crushed rosemary

½ teaspoon salt

1 teaspoon coarsely ground pepper

1 cup beef stock

½ cup cooking liquid from roast

1 lb Portobello mushrooms, sliced thin

1 tablespoon Vermouth

1. Rinse the heart with cold water and pat dry.

2. Combine olive oil, balsamic vinegar, pressed garlic, rosemary, salt and pepper in a bowl. Add the heart and turn to coat liberally with the mixture.

3. Place the heart in the slow cooker. Add the beef stock. Cover and cook on Low for 6 to 8 hours or on High for 3 to 4 hours until meat is very tender. During the last half hour of cooking, take ½ cup of the cooking liquid from the slow cooker and put it in a skillet. Heat on medium, and add the mushrooms. Cook, stirring, until they begin to soften, about 3 minutes. Turn heat to low and simmer, covered, stirring occasionally, until mushrooms are soft, about 20 to 30 minutes.

4. Turn heat to high, and when mushrooms are hot, add the Vermouth and stir. Stand back slightly and strike a match over the mushroom mix. The alcohol will catch fire. Shake the pan until the flames subside. Serve the warm mushrooms with slices of the meat.

A healthy heart is slightly pink in color and has a nice layer of fat on it. Your local farmer or butcher will know how to prepare it, but it's best with some of the fat left on.

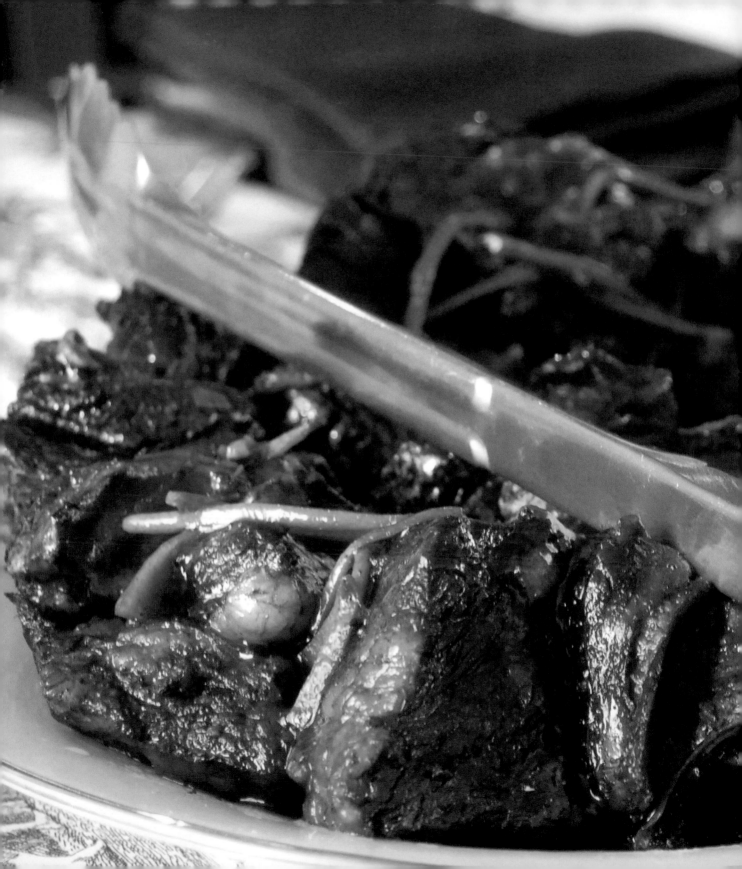

Short Ribs of Beef with Rosemary and Fennel

Short ribs are a wonderful cut because they become so meltingly tender when slowly braised in the slow cooker. The aromatic rosemary in the simple sauce cuts through the richness of the meat well.

Makes 4 to 6 servings.

5 pounds meaty short ribs with bones

¼ cup olive oil

1 large onion, minced

4 cloves of garlic, sliced

2 cups beef stock or broth

1 large fennel bulb, cored, trimmed, and sliced

2 tablespoons fresh rosemary

2 tablespoons fresh parsley, chopped

2 teaspoons arrowroot

Salt and pepper to taste

1. Preheat the oven broiler, and line a broiler pan with heavy-duty aluminum foil. Broil short ribs for 3 to 4 minutes per side, or until browned. Arrange short ribs in the slow cooker, and pour in any juices that have collected in the pan.

2. Heat oil in a medium skillet over medium-high heat. Add onion and garlic, and cook, stirring frequently, for 3 minutes, or until onion is translucent. Scrape mixture into the slow cooker. Add stock, fennel, parsley, and rosemary to the slow cooker, and stir well.

3. Cook on Low for 8 to 10 hours or on High for 4 to 5 hours, or until short ribs are very tender. Remove as much grease as possible from the slow cooker with a soup ladle.

4. If cooking on Low, raise the heat to High. Mix arrowroot with 2 tablespoons cold water in a small cup. Stir this mixture into the cooker, and cook on High for 15 to 20 minutes, or until juices are bubbling and slightly thickened. Season with salt and pepper.

Our English word for beef comes from the Latin *bos,* which means "ox." By the Middle Ages, it had become *boef* or beef in English. There were cattle at the Jamestown settlement in Virginia in the early seventeenth century, but the Texas longhorns that we use for beef today were brought to that state by the Spanish almost a century after the Jamestown settlement.

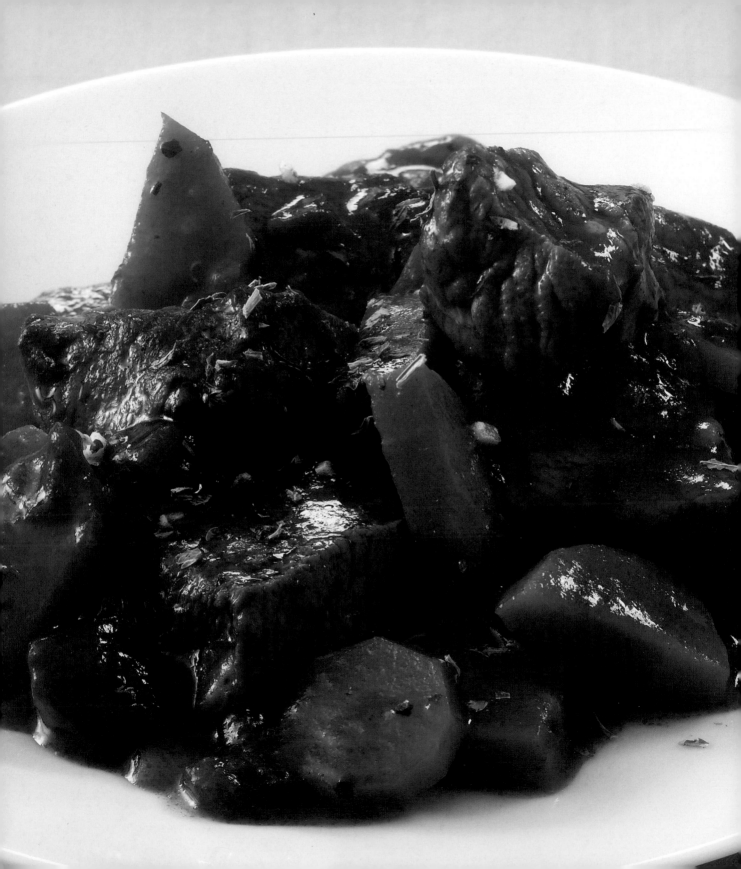

Classic Veal Stew

This is an elegant and simple combination of tomatoes and peas that create a delectable sauce to accompany the tender veal.

Makes 4 to 6 servings.

1 tablespoon olive oil

2 tablespoons ghee

1 to 2 pounds veal shoulder or shank, cubed

Almond flour (approximately ½ cup)

1 small onion, chopped

1 8-oz can diced tomatoes, with the juice

1 10-oz package frozen baby Brussels sprouts

Salt and pepper

1. Put the oil and 1 tablespoon of the ghee in a heavy-bottomed skillet. In a shallow bowl or on a plate, put a layer of almond flour. Dust the veal cubes with the flour, setting them aside when coated. Heat the oil and ghee to high, and add the flour-dusted cubes, stirring, so that the meat browns on all sides. Work in batches if necessary. As the batches of cubes are browned, transfer them to the slow cooker.

2. Heat the additional tablespoon of ghee in the skillet and add the onion, stirring until the bits are translucent, about 3 minutes. Add the tomatoes, stir, and transfer this to the slow cooker over the meat.

3. Cover and cook on Low for 5 to 6 hours or on High for 3 to 4 hours. Add the frozen Brussels sprouts. Continue to cook on Low for another 1 to 2 hours, or on High for another 30 to 60 minutes. Season with salt and pepper when cooked.

Variation:

This stew could be prepared with additional vegetables if desired. You could add fresh asparagus cut into inch-sized pieces, baby mushrooms, even a cup or so of cubed squash. Give them time to cook with the meat and the tomato sauce to reach their fullest flavor.

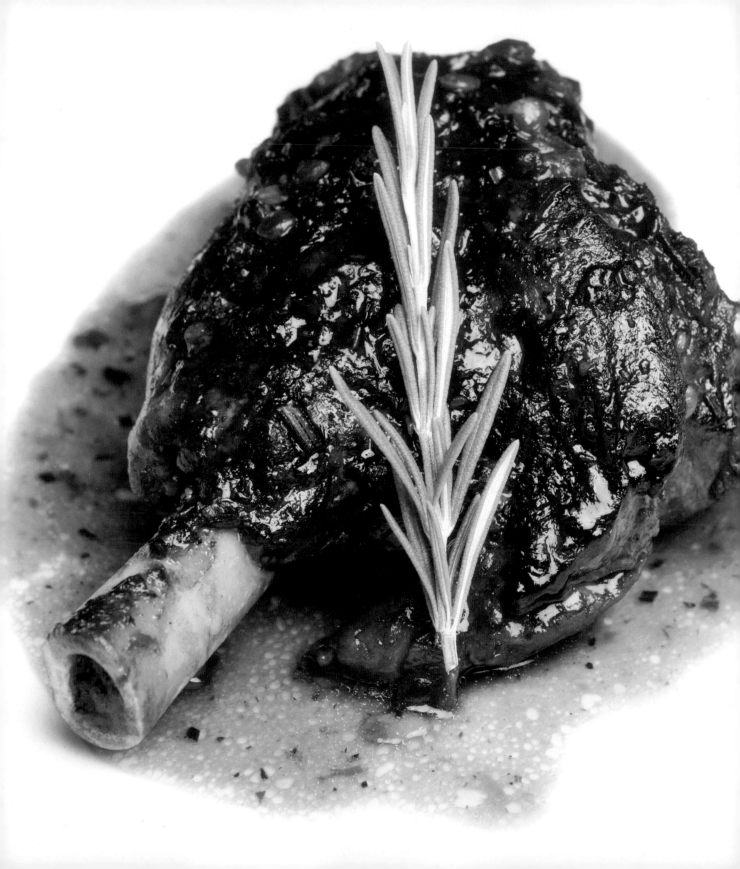

Lamb Shanks with Olives and Artichoke Hearts

While "white meats" are frequently cooked in red wine, it's unusual for red meats to be cooked in white wine. But that's the basis of this dish, punctuated by salty black olives and delicate artichoke hearts.

Makes 4 to 6 servings.

4 to 6 (12- to 14-oz) lamb shanks

3 tablespoons olive oil

1 large onion, chopped

3 cloves garlic, minced

1 cup beef stock or broth

2 ripe tomatoes, seeded and chopped, with juice, or 1 8-oz can tomato sauce

1 cup dry white wine

2 tablespoons fresh rosemary, chopped

2 tablespoons fresh parsley, chopped

12 baby artichokes, trimmed with outer leaves removed, and halved

½ cup pitted black oil-cured olives

1 tablespoon arrowroot

Salt and pepper to taste

1. Preheat the oven broiler, and line a broiler pan with heavy-duty aluminum foil. Broil lamb shanks for 3 minutes per side, or until browned. Transfer lamb to the slow cooker, and pour in any juices that have collected in the pan.

2. Heat oil in a medium skillet over medium-high heat. Add onion and garlic, and cook, stirring frequently, for 3 minutes, or until onion is translucent. Scrape mixture into the slow cooker. Add stock, tomato sauce, wine, rosemary, and parsley to the slow cooker, and stir well.

3. Cook shanks on Low for 6 to 8 hours or on High for 3 to 4 hours, or until lamb is almost tender. Add artichokes and olives to the slow cooker, and cook for 2 hours on Low or 1 hour on High.

4. If cooking on Low, raise the heat to High. Mix arrowroot with 2 tablespoons cold water in a small cup. Add this mixture to the slow cooker, cover, and cook for an additional 10 to 15 minutes, or until the juices are bubbling and slightly thickened. Season with salt and pepper to taste.

Like apples and avocados, artichokes darken when exposed to air. When preparing them, have a bowl of cold water acidulated with lemon juice on the counter. Drop the artichokes into it as you trim the stems and pull off the outer leaves.

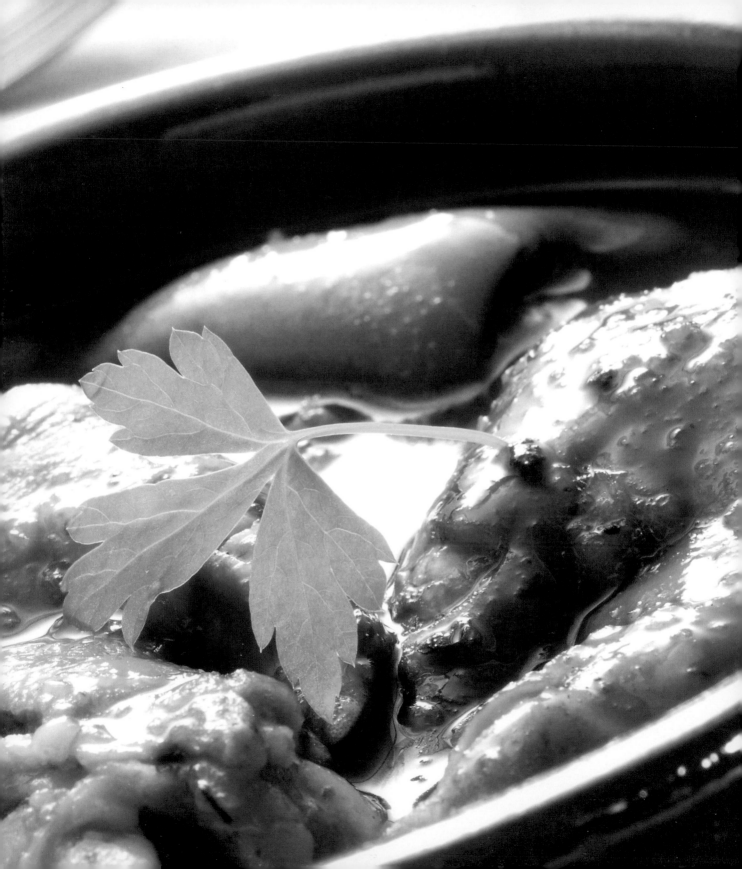

Slow-Roasted Pigs' Feet

If you thought this was a cut that was only served deep-fried, guess again! With the traditional Italian accompaniments of tomatoes, garlic, and basil, what might seem like a down-and-dirty cut of meat is transformed into a delectable, tender, concoction resembling pulled pork.

Makes 4 to 6 servings.

6 pigs' feet, halved and quartered by your farmer or butcher

Salt and pepper

3 tablespoons olive oil

1 onion, chopped

2 cloves garlic, minced

4 fresh basil leaves, shredded

Two 14.5-oz cans diced tomatoes, with sauce

1. Wash and pat dry the pigs' feet. Season with salt and pepper. Set aside.

2. In a skillet over medium heat, add olive oil and onions. Cook, stirring, until onions are translucent, about three minutes. Add the garlic and stir for another minute. Transfer the mixture to the slow cooker. Add the shredded basil.

3. Place the pigs' feet on top of the onion mixture, and add the tomatoes. Cover and cook on Low for 10 to 12 hours or on High for 8 to 10 hours, until the meat is falling from the bone.

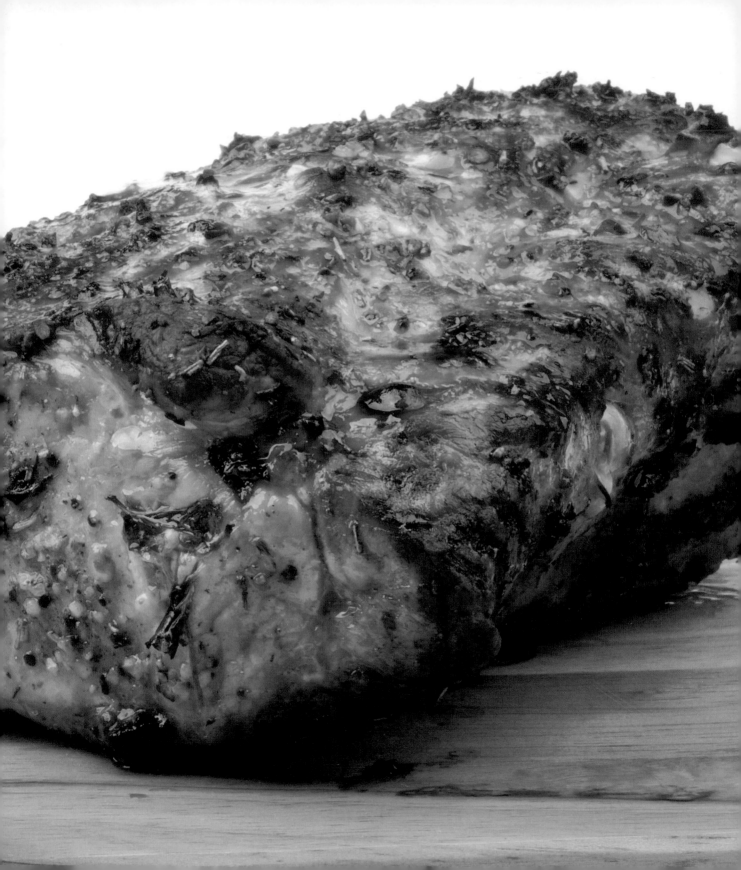

Herbed Pork Roast

Pork is a best friend of garlic, and this recipe calls for plenty of it! Between that and the fresh herbs, by the time this dish is cooked, everyone's mouths will be watering from the aroma.

Makes 6 to 8 servings.

2-pound boneless pork roast

6 cloves garlic, minced

¼ cup fresh rosemary, chopped

2 tablespoons fresh parsley, chopped

2 tablespoons fresh sage, chopped

Salt and pepper to taste

3 ribs celery, cut into 4-inch lengths

⅓ cup chicken stock or broth

1. Rinse pork and pat dry with paper towels. Combine garlic, rosemary, parsley, sage, salt, and pepper in a mixing bowl. Make slits deep in the pork, and stuff half of mixture into the slits. Rub remaining mixture on the outside of the roast.

2. Arrange celery slices in the bottom of the slow cooker to form a bed for the meat.

3. Preheat the oven broiler, and line a broiler pan with heavy-duty aluminum foil. Broil pork for 3 minutes per side, until well browned. Transfer port to the slow cooker, and pour in any juices that have collected in the pan. Pour stock over pork.

4. Cover and cook on High for about 2 hours, then reduce heat to Low and cook for 4 hours, until pork is fork tender. Carve pork into slices and moisten with juices from the slow cooker.

Browning meat under the broiler accomplishes two things when using a slow cooker. It gives the meat a more appealing color, and it heats it so that it passes through the "danger zone" of 40F to 140F faster, especially if you're cooking on Low.

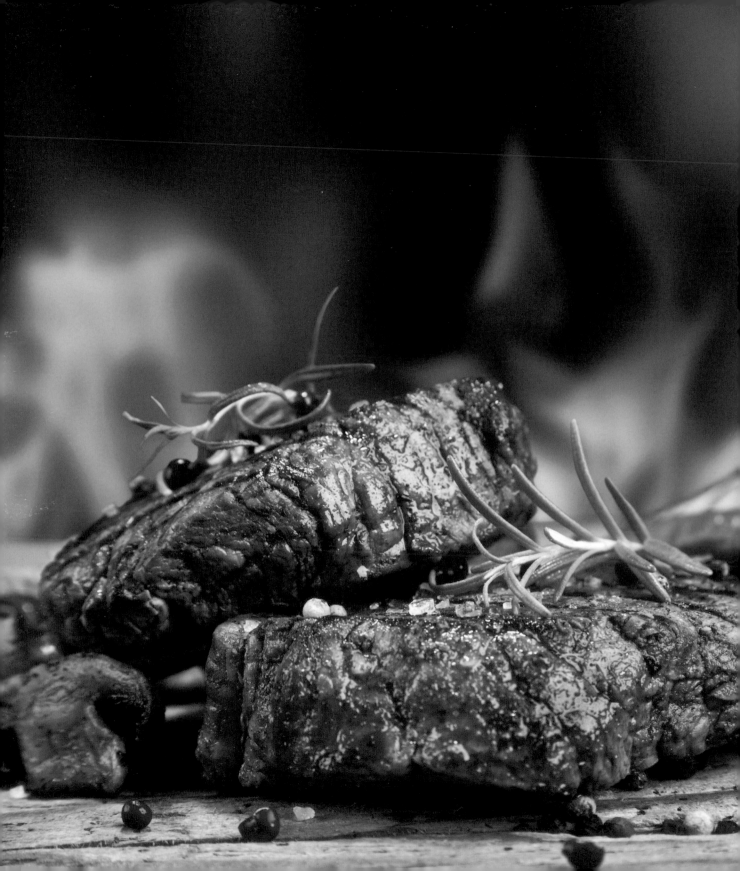

Roast Heart to Fall in Love With

Take advantage of the steak-like quality of a heart. Remember that it's an organ loaded with lots of nutrients, and when you cook it as you would a rump roast, you will have a power-packed, super-delicious meal—and possibly some tasty leftovers.

Makes 4 to 6 servings.

2- to 3-pound beef heart

3 tablespoons olive oil

1 large onion, diced

4 cloves garlic, minced

2 cups beef stock or broth

4 ribs celery, trimmed and cut into slices

3 carrots, sliced

2 tablespoons fresh rosemary, chopped

2 tablespoons fresh parsley, chopped

1 teaspoon fresh thyme, chopped

1½ tablespoons arrowroot

Salt and pepper to taste

1. Cut the heart in half and remove any tough parts. Preheat the oven broiler, and line a broiler pan with heavy-duty aluminum foil. Broil the heart for 2 to 3 minutes per side, or until browned. Transfer the heart to the slow cooker, and pour in any juices that have collected in the pan.

2. Heat oil in a medium skillet over medium-high heat. Add onion and garlic and cook, stirring frequently, for 3 minutes, or until onion is translucent. Scrape mixture into the slow cooker.

3. Add stock, celery, carrots, rosemary, and thyme to the slow cooker, and stir well. Cook on Low for 8 to 10 hours or on High for 4 to 5 hours, or until the meat is very tender.

4. If cooking on Low, raise the heat to High. Mix arrowroot with 2 tablespoons cold water in a small cup, and stir it into the slow cooker. Cook on High for 15 to 20 minutes, or until juices are bubbling and slightly thickened.

5. Remove roast from the slow cooker. Season to taste with salt and pepper. Slice into thin slices and serve the vegetables and juices on the side. Garnish with some additional parsley if desired.

While roasted meats need time to "rest" during which the juices are reabsorbed into the fibers of the meat, that is not necessary for braised dishes. The juices from the meat are integrated into the sauce, which then moistens the meat.

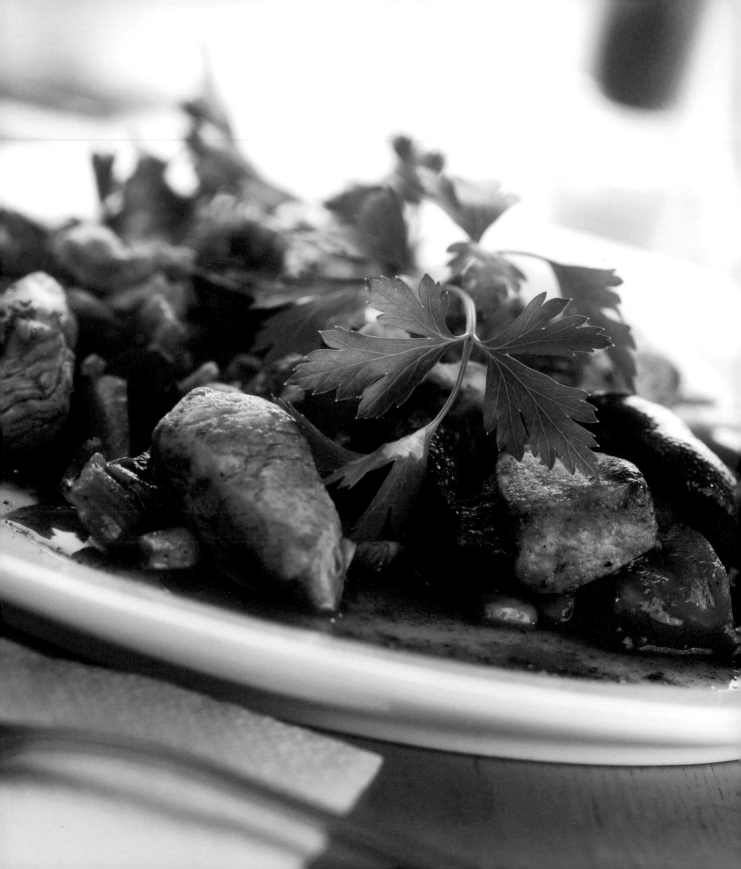

Mediterranean Pork Stew

This vibrant stew punctuated with olives contains many of the flavors common to dishes traditionally found along the Mediterranean coast, including red bell peppers and leeks. *Mangia!*

Makes 6 to 8 servings.

1½ pounds boneless pork loin, cut into cubes

4 leeks, white parts only

2 juice oranges, washed

2 tablespoons coconut oil

4 cloves garlic, minced

2 red bell peppers, seeds and ribs removed, and thinly sliced

14.5-oz can diced tomatoes, drained

1 cup dry red wine

1 cup chicken stock or broth

¾ cup pitted oil-cured black olives

3 tablespoons fresh parsley, chopped

1 teaspoon thyme

1 teaspoon oregano

1 bay leaf

1 tablespoon arrowroot

Salt and pepper to taste

1. Preheat the oven broiler, and line a broiler pan with heavy-duty aluminum foil. Broil pork for 3 minutes per side, or until browned. Transfer cubes to the slow cooker, and pour in any juices that have collected in the pan.

2. Trim leeks, split lengthwise, and slice thinly. Place slices in a colander and rinse well under cold running water, rubbing with your fingers to dislodge all dirt. Shake leeks in the colander. Grate zest from oranges and squeeze juice from oranges. Set aside.

3. Heat oil in a medium skillet over medium-high heat. Add leeks, garlic, and red peppers, and cook, stirring frequently, for 3 minutes, or until leeks are translucent. Scrape mixture into the slow cooker.

4. Add tomatoes, orange juice and zest, wine, stock, olives, parsley, thyme, oregano, and bay leaf to the slow cooker, and stir well. Cook on Low for 6 to 8 hours or on High for 3 to 4 hours, or until pork is tender.

5. If cooking on Low, raise the heat to High. Mix arrowroot with 2 tablespoons cold water in a small cup, and stir it into the slow cooker. Cook on High for 15 to 20 minutes, or until juices are bubbling and slightly thickened. Remove and discard bay leaf, and season to taste with salt and pepper.

> **Pitted olives may be more intention than reality. That's why it's always worth the time to look over pitted olives carefully and not just dump them into a pot. More than one dentist has been called late at night because a patient bit down on an olive to discover a molar-cracking pit.**

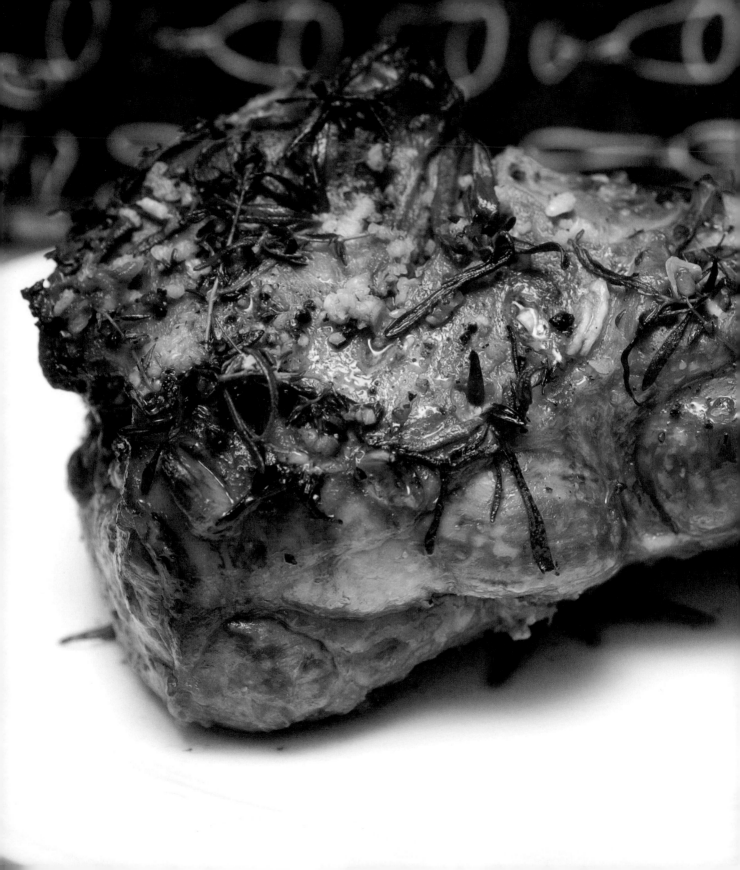

Leg of Lamb with Rosemary

For Italians, roast lamb symbolizes spring and rebirth. It is the traditional dish of Easter. Shop like your Nonna for this recipe and ask your local farmer for a shoulder of spring lamb.

Makes 4 to 6 servings.

Spring lamb shoulder roast, about 2½ pounds

1 tablespoon olive oil

½ teaspoon sea salt

½ teaspoon freshly ground black pepper

1 teaspoon fresh rosemary, chopped

3 cloves garlic, minced

½ cup dry white wine

1. Wash and pat dry the lamb. Put the olive oil in your hands and rub the oil all over the lamb.

2. Put the lamb in the slow cooker and sprinkle it all over with the salt, pepper, rosemary, and garlic, rubbing the spices onto the meat. Add the wine to the slow cooker.

3. Cover and cook on Low for 8 to 10 hours or until very tender. Do not cook on High. Season with additional salt and pepper if desired.

Italians turn to other fresh spring ingredients for their Easter celebrations. Pair this delicious roast with spring peas or asparagus or a salad of new spring greens.

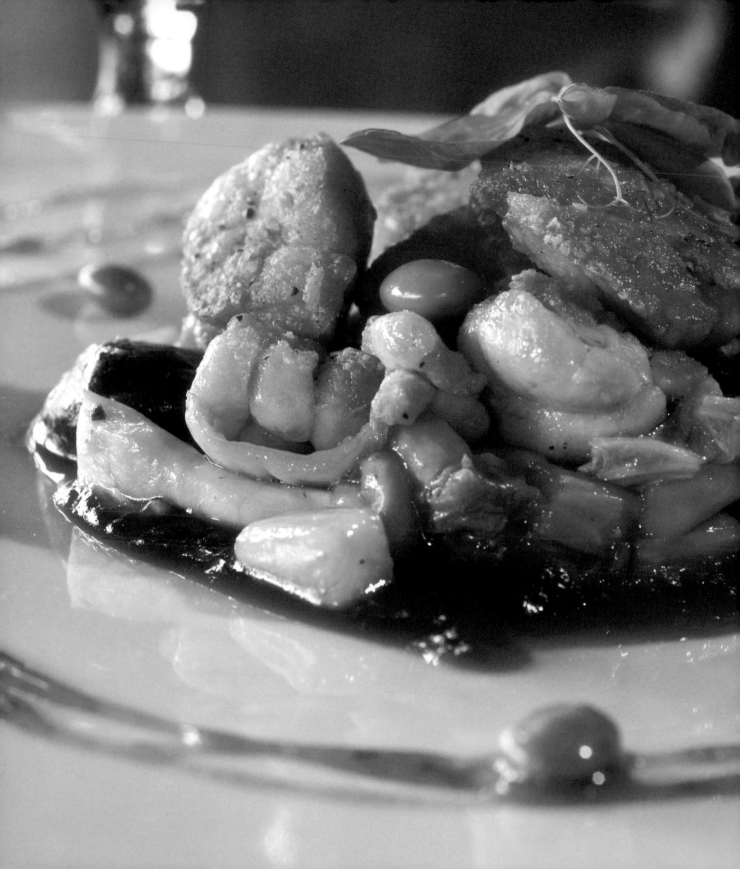

Vegetable-Infused Sweetbreads

All of the ancient cuisines featured recipes using organ meats and other "offal." How the thymus gland of young cows, pigs, and sheep came to be known as "sweetbreads" is somewhat of a mystery, but so be it. Sweetbreads are considered a delicacy in some parts of the world. This recipe calls for veal or calf sweetbreads, which are more tender than those from other animals. The texture is a bit like gnocchi. As some cooks say, "Who needs to know what it is as long as it tastes good?" Try this one and see if you have otherwise reticent eaters coming back for more.

Makes 6 to 8 servings.

3 pounds veal sweetbreads (about 6 pieces)

Cold water to cover

1 teaspoon salt

Salt and pepper

2 tablespoons olive oil

1 tablespoon walnut oil

8 shallots, sliced

2 leeks, white parts only, sliced and washed

2 carrots, sliced thin

1 stalk celery, chopped

1 tablespoon peppercorns

3 cups chicken stock, warmed

Fresh parsley for garnish

1. Start a day early. Soak the sweetbreads in cold water to cover into which a teaspoon of salt has been added. After 6 to 8 hours, remove and discard the water. Remove any membranes. Put the sweetbreads on a plate, cover with another plate, and put a heavy bowl on top. Press them between the plates until ready to cook. Season the pressed sweetbreads pieces with salt and pepper on both sides.

2. Heat the olive and walnut oils in a skillet over medium-high heat. Add the sweetbreads and brown on both sides, about 25 seconds a side. Transfer browned meat to a plate. Into the remaining oil, add the shallots, leeks, carrots, and celery. Cook, stirring, until vegetables are just softening, about 3 minutes. Transfer the mix to the slow cooker, including the oil in the pan. Add the peppercorns.

3. Place the sweetbreads over the vegetable mixture. Pour the warmed stock over everything. Cover and cook on Low for 4 to 6 hours or on High for 1½ to 2½ hours.

4. Put the cooked sweetbreads on a platter and cover to keep warm. Puree the vegetable mix with an immersion blender or by processing in a blender. Pour the vegetable sauce over the sweetbreads. Drizzle with some additional walnut oil, if desired, and garnish with parsley.

While sweetbreads are neither sweet nor bready, they are loaded with protein and calories. A 4-ounce serving has nearly twice as many calories as a similar portion of sirloin steak. According to the website Livestrong, "...it would take 42 minutes of swimming laps or one hour and 39 minutes of weightlifting..." to burn the 360 calories contained in that small portion size.

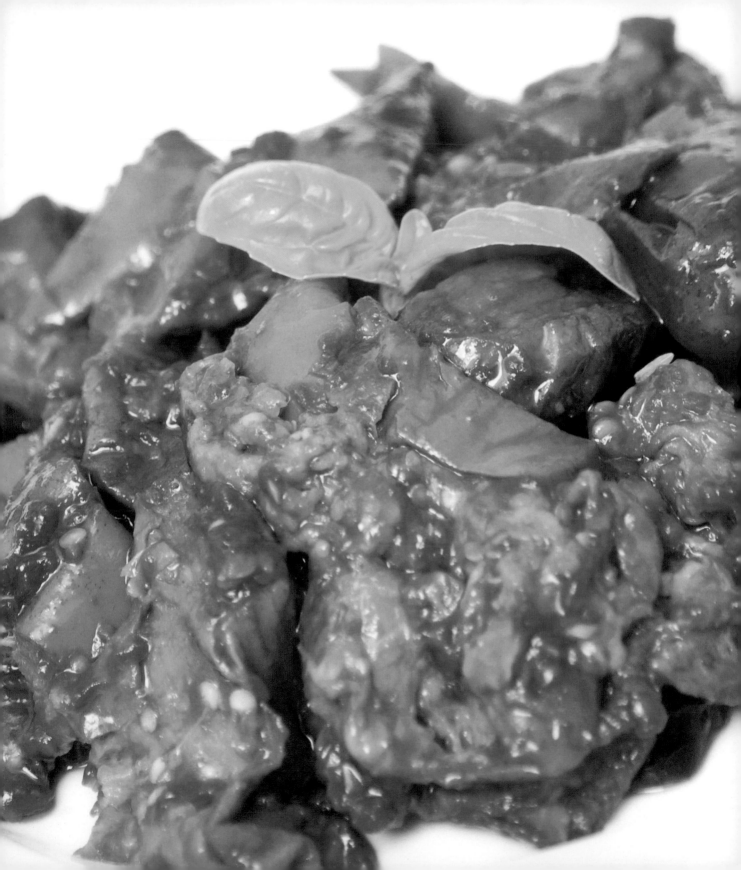

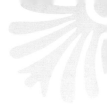

Lamb and Eggplant Stew

The tomatoes, eggplant, zucchini, and garlic provide a ratatouille base to the succulent lamb in this wonderful late-summer stew. Using a large quantity of bay leaves is a Turkish influence.

Makes 4 to 6 servings.

1½ pounds boneless leg of lamb, cubed

½ teaspoon salt

½ teaspoon pepper

1½ tablespoons olive oil

2 large onions, thinly sliced

5 cloves garlic, minced

14-oz can diced tomatoes, undrained

1 eggplant, cut into thick slices

1 zucchini, cut into thick slices

4 bay leaves

3 tablespoons fresh parsley chopped

1. Sprinkle the salt and pepper on the chunks of lamb. Heat the oil in a skillet over medium-high heat and add the chunks, working in batches to brown the meat on all sides, about 3 minutes a batch. As the chunks are browned, transfer to the slow cooker.

2. To the same skillet, add a little more oil, and add the onions and garlic, stirring to cook for about 3 minutes, until the onions are translucent. Add the mix to the slow cooker.

3. Add the tomatoes, eggplant, zucchini, and bay leaves. Cover and cook on Low for 6 to 8 hours or on High for 4 to 5 hours, until lamb is tender. Add parsley, stir to combine, and cook for another 10 minutes.

Bay leaves—a key ingredient to most stew recipes—are dried leaves from bay laurel trees. They originated in Asia Minor, most notably Turkey, and spread to other areas that were warm enough to cultivate them. They have been a culinary staple since recorded history, and figure prominently in the history and mythology of ancient Rome. The dried leaves lend a mild but distinct flavor reminiscent of thyme, but more subtle and deep.

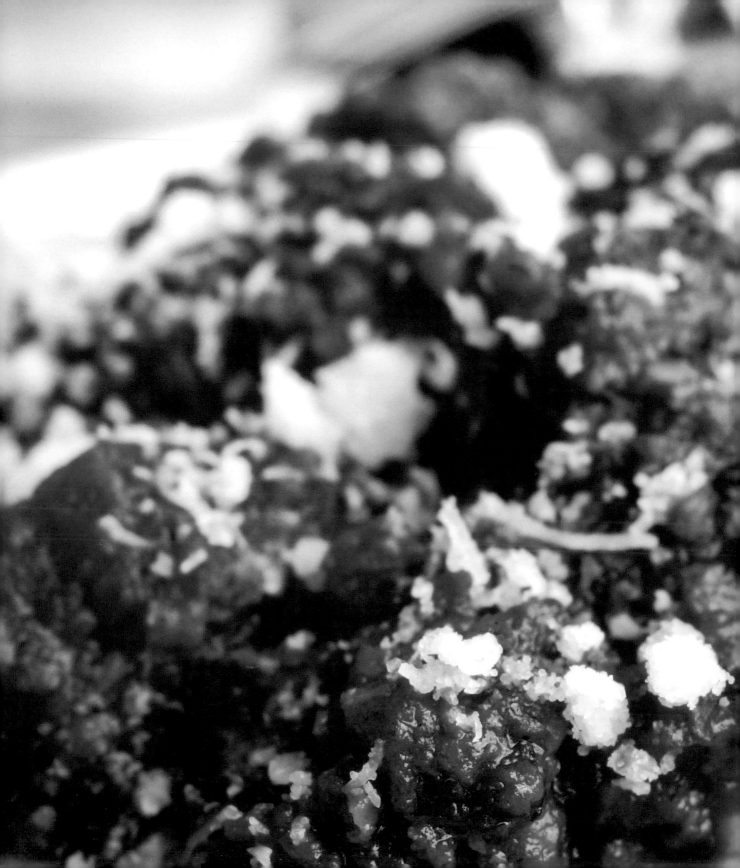

Beef and Sausage Ragu

The sausage adds some additional fat and flavor to this irresistible dish. It might not meet with your Italian in-laws' approval, but it'll be quickly devoured by all.

Makes 6 to 8 servings.

1 tablespoon olive oil

1 onion, chopped

1 pound ground beef

1 pound Italian sweet sausage, casing removed

Three 28-oz cans tomato puree

5 cloves garlic, minced

2 tablespoons fresh parsley, chopped fine

3 bay leaves

1 teaspoon dried oregano

1 teaspoon crushed red pepper flakes (optional)

Salt and pepper

1. In a large skillet, heat the oil and add the onion. Cook, stirring, until onion is translucent, about 3 minutes. Add the ground meats and continue to cook, stirring, breaking up the sausage meat while both meats brown. Only cook partially until meat just loses its pink color, about 2 minutes.

2. Transfer the meat mixture to the slow cooker. In the skillet, put the tomato puree, garlic, parsley, bay leaves, oregano, and red pepper flakes. Stir and heat to warm.

3. Add the tomato mixture over the ground meats and onions. Cover and cook on Low for 8 to 10 hours or on High for 5 to 7 hours. Season with salt and pepper to taste.

Variations:

* If you want the mix to be extra spicy, use hot Italian sausage instead of sweet sausage, and increase the amount of crushed red pepper to your liking.
* For a Paleo-appropriate side that will satisfy like pasta, prepare some cauliflower "rice" by chopping cauliflower florets into rice-sized pieces and sautéing in ghee until just tender. Season with salt, pepper, and parsley if desired.

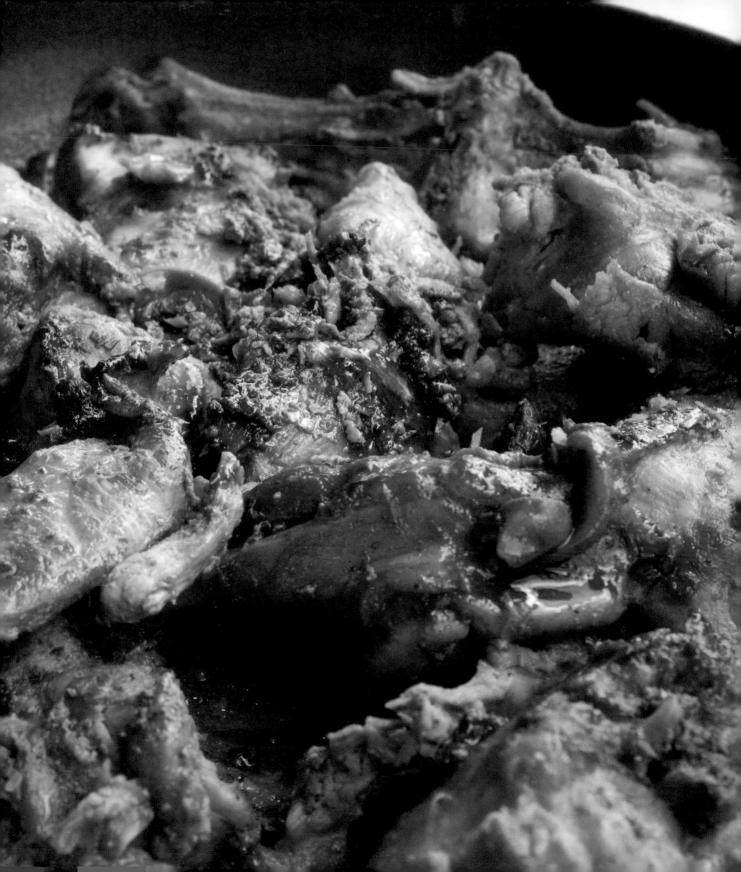

Rabbit Stew

Rabbit is a readily available meat for people who live in the country. In many places, you can find it at farmer's markets, which is a great source for fresh meat.

Makes 4 to 6 servings.

1 tablespoon olive oil

2 tablespoons ghee

1 to 2 pounds rabbit pieces

Almond flour (approximately ½ cup)

2 leeks, white parts only, sliced thin and washed thoroughly

1 stalk celery, sliced thin

Two 8-oz cans diced tomatoes, with the juice

Salt and pepper

1. Put the oil and 1 tablespoon of the ghee in a heavy-bottomed skillet. In a shallow bowl or on a plate, put a layer of almond flour. Dust the rabbit pieces with the flour, setting them aside when coated. Heat the oil and ghee to high, and add the flour-dusted cubes, stirring, so that the meat browns on all sides. Work in batches if necessary. As the batches of cubes are browned, transfer them to the slow cooker.

2. Heat the additional tablespoon of ghee in the skillet and add the leeks and celery, stirring until the bits are translucent, about 5 minutes. Add the tomatoes, stir, and transfer this to the slow cooker over the meat.

3. Cover and cook on Low for 6 to 8 hours or on High for 4 to 5 hours. Season with salt and pepper when cooked.

> Rabbit is a delicious meat source that has been eaten by our ancestors for millennia. But it's hard not to think of rabbits as cute and soft and cuddly. They are. And so are deer, and cows, and pigs, and sheep. One thing about committing to this diet as that you need to make your peace with meat.

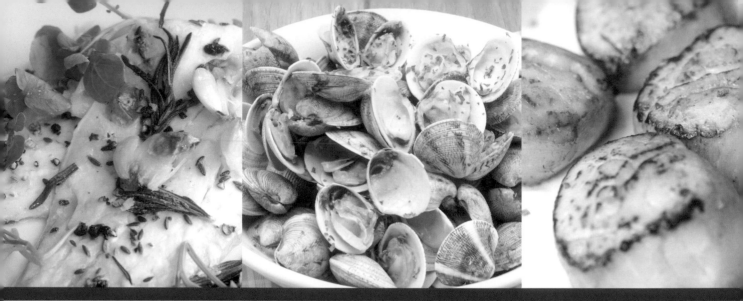

Chapter 7

Paleo *Secondi:*

Fish and Seafood

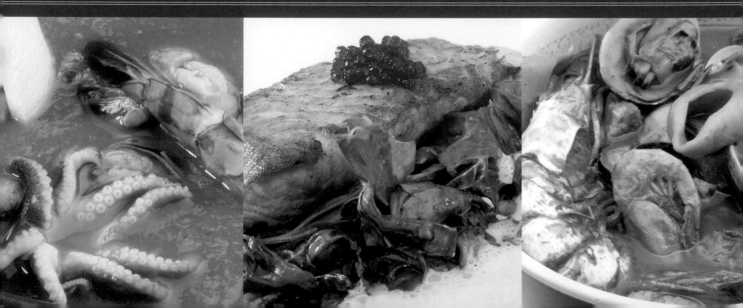

With Italy's extensive coastlines, it's no wonder fish feature prominently in the country's cuisine. The secret to sensational dishes rests on the simple premise of fresh, high-quality ingredients. There is nothing tastier than a fresh filet of brook trout, seasoned with hints of salt and pepper, and steamed in its own juice with a hint of lemon. Paleo eaters will want to incorporate lots of fresh fish into an otherwise meat-based diet; doing this is not only nutritionally sound, but offers taste treats you might not otherwise have explored.

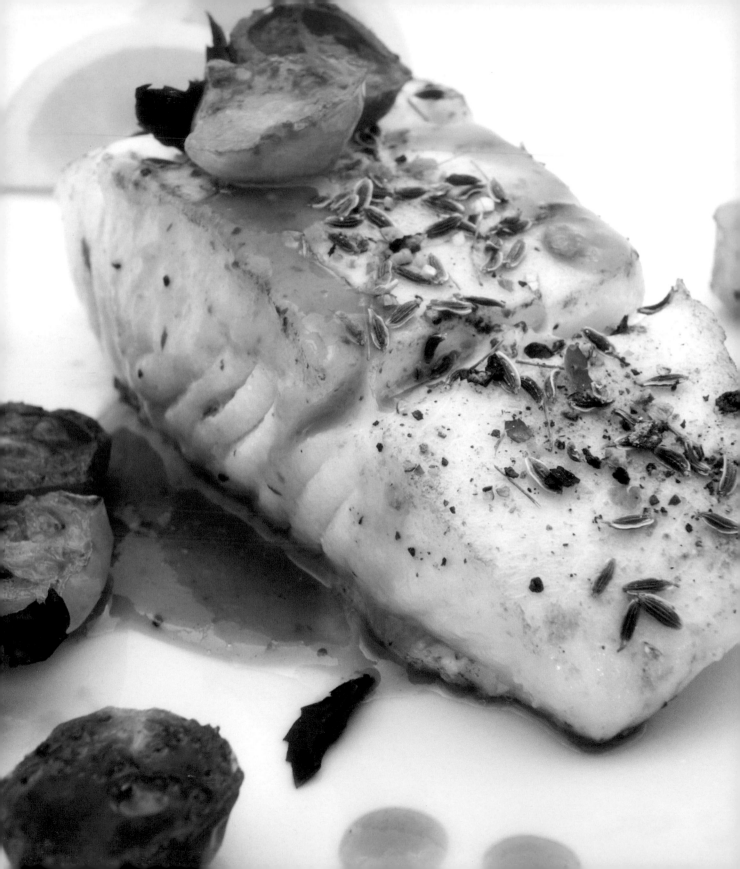

Fish with Tomatoes and Fennel

In this colorful dish, fish fillets are cooked on top of a delicious and aromatic bed of vegetables scented with orange. Close your eyes and pretend you're dining on the Italian coast.

Makes 4 to 6 servings.

2 medium fennel bulbs

¼ cup olive oil

1 large onion, thinly sliced

2 cloves garlic, minced

28-oz can diced tomatoes, drained

1 tablespoon grated orange zest

½ cup freshly squeezed orange juice

1 tablespoon fennel seeds, crushed

2 pounds thick, firm-fleshed fish fillets (such as cod, halibut, or tilapia), cut into serving-sized pieces

Salt and pepper to taste

1. Discard stalks from fennel, and save for another use. Rinse fennel, cut in half lengthwise, and discard core and top layer of flesh. Slice fennel thinly and set aside.

2. Heat oil in a large skillet over medium-high heat. Add onion and garlic, and cook, stirring frequently, for 3 minutes, or until onion is translucent. Add fennel and cook for an additional 2 minutes. Scrape mixture into the slow cooker.

3. Add tomatoes, zest, orange juice, and fennel seeds to the slow cooker. Stir well to combine. Cook on Low for 5 to 7 hours, or on High for 2 to 3 hours, or until fennel is crisp-tender.

4. If cooking on Low, raise the heat to High. Season fish with salt and pepper, and place it on top of vegetables. Cover and cook for 30 to 45 minutes, or until fish is cooked through and flakes easily. Season to taste with salt and pepper.

The vegetable mixture can be cooked up to 2 days in advance and refrigerated, tightly covered. Reheat it in a microwave oven or over low heat, and return it to the slow cooker. Increase the heat to High and cook the fish just prior to serving, as described above.

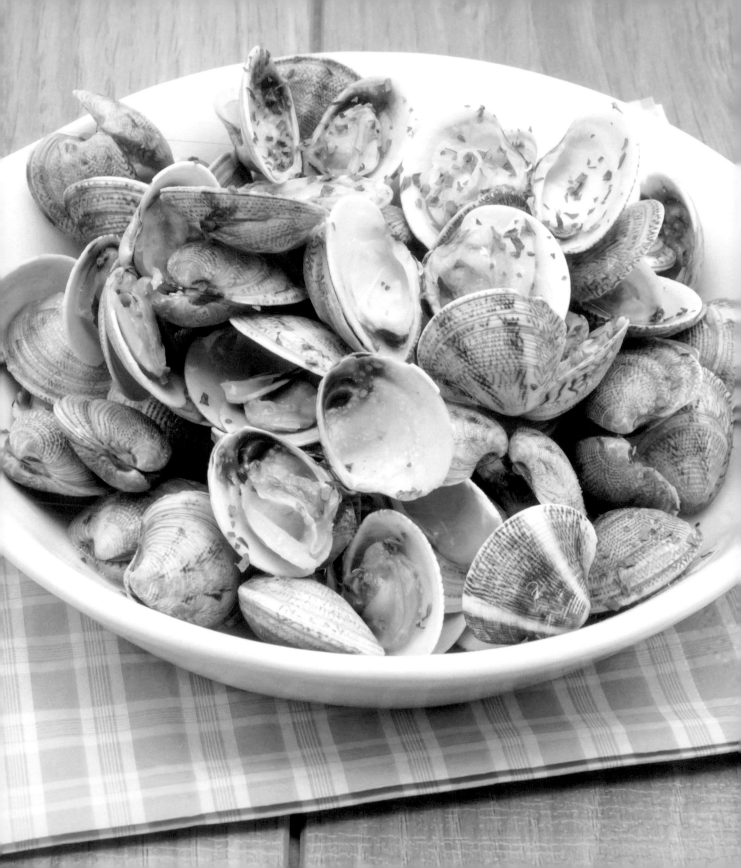

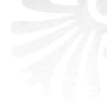

Clams with Pesto

Basil is a lovely fresh herb to accompany shellfish. This is a dish that showcases summer's bounty—fresh clams, fresh basil, even fresh garlic.

Makes 4 to 6 servings.

Makes 2 to 4 servings.

3 dozen littleneck clams, rinsed

1 cup dry white wine

1 cup fresh basil leaves (packed full)

⅓ cup walnut pieces

3 cloves garlic, minced;

¼ cup olive oil

Salt and pepper to taste.

1. Place the wine with the clams in the slow cooker. Cover and cook on High, taking a look every 20 to 30 minutes to see how the clams are opening up. Stir the clams to ensure heat distribution for proper opening.

2. While the clams are cooking, prepare the pesto. Using a food processor, put the basil leaves, walnut pieces and garlic in the bowl and pulse until all is chopped. Stream in the olive oil while continuing to pulse until you have a nice consistency.

3. When clams are open, transfer them to a large serving bowl. Pour the clam/wine juice into another bowl, being careful to let any sand stay in the slow cooker. Add the pesto to the clam sauce, and pour over the cooked clams.

Variations:

Pesto can be made with different kinds of nuts and herbs.

✳ Use flat leaf parsley instead of basil.

✳ Use pine nuts instead of walnuts.

✳ Use unsalted cashews instead of walnuts.

> Pesto freezes well, so you may want to double this recipe and put half aside for future use. Because a little goes a long way, try freezing it in an ice cube tray.

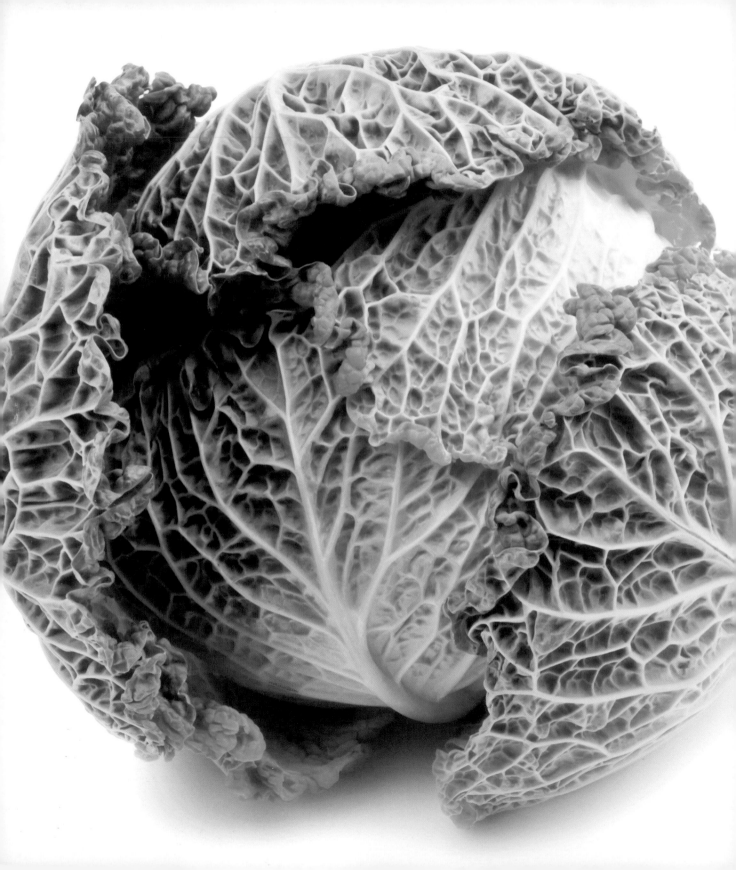

Monkfish with Cabbage, Pancetta, and Rosemary

Monkfish, sometimes called "poor man's lobster" because its sweet flavor and texture are similar to the prized crustacean, is popular in the regions bordering the Adriatic Sea in Italy.

Makes 4 to 6 servings.

½ small (1½ pounds) head Savoy or green cabbage

¼ pound pancetta, diced

2 pounds monkfish fillets, trimmed and cut into serving pieces

2 cloves garlic, minced

1 cup fish stock or broth

2 tablespoons fresh rosemary, chopped, or 2 teaspoons dried

1 tablespoon fresh parsley, chopped

2 teaspoons grated lemon zest

Salt and pepper to taste

1 tablespoon fresh parsley, chopped

1. Rinse and core cabbage. Cut into wedges and then shred cabbage. Bring a large pot of salted water to a boil. Add cabbage and boil for 4 minutes. Drain cabbage and place it in the slow cooker.

2. Cook pancetta in a heavy skillet over medium heat for 5 to 7 minutes, or until crisp. Remove pancetta from the skillet with a slotted spoon, and place it in the slow cooker. Raise the heat to high, and sear the monkfish in the fat on all sides, turning the pieces gently with tongs, until browned. Refrigerate fish.

3. Add garlic, stock, rosemary, parsley, and lemon zest to the slow cooker, and stir well. Cook on Low for 3 to 4 hours or on High for 1 to 2 hours, or until cabbage is almost tender.

4. If cooking on Low, raise the heat to High. Season monkfish with salt and pepper, and place it on top of the vegetables. Cook monkfish for 30 to 45 minutes, or until it is cooked through. Remove monkfish from the slow cooker, and keep it warm. Season the cabbage with salt and pepper.

5. To serve, mound equal-sized portions of cabbage on each plate. Slice monkfish into medallions and arrange on top of cabbage. Garnish with fresh parsley.

> Cabbage is clearly one of the sturdier vegetables, and it will keep refrigerated for up to six weeks if not cut. Looser heads like Savoy and Napa cabbage should be used within three weeks. Do not wash it before storing, because moisture will bring on decay.

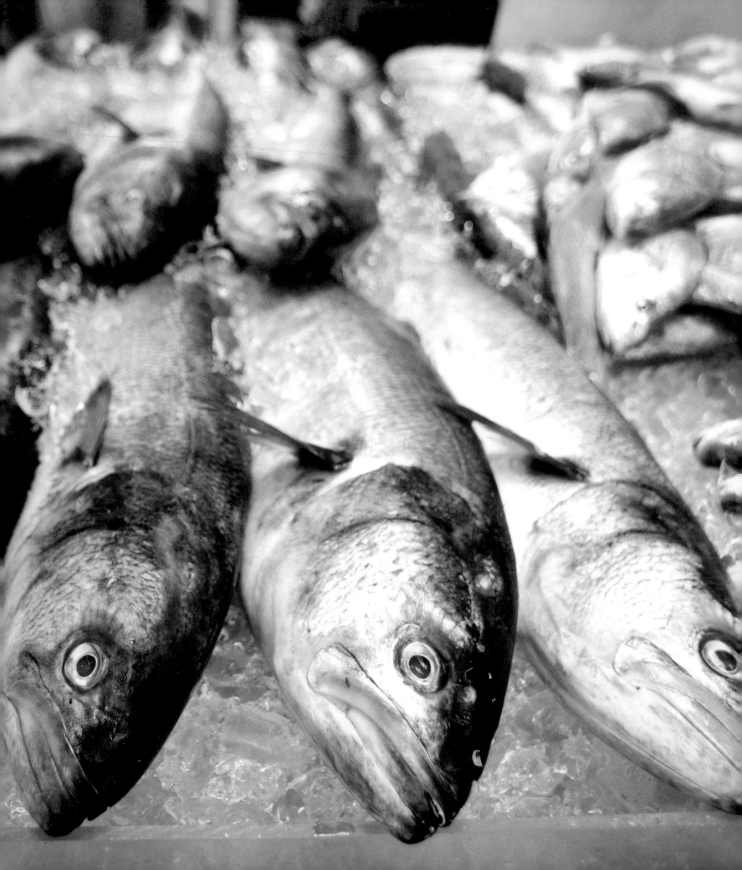

Lemon-Tarragon Bluefish

Bluefish is one that people either love or hate. It's considered an oily fish, and it has an almost gamey taste. It's found all around the world, so it's a fish that has sustained us for millennia. Paleo appropriate!

Makes 4 to 6 servings.

3 pounds bluefish fillet

2 tablespoons fresh tarragon, chopped

2 lemons

1 large onion, thinly sliced

Salt and pepper to taste

1. Make sure the fillets are free of bones. Put them skin side down into the slow cooker. Sprinkle the tarragon over the fish, then squeeze the lemons over them. Remove any seeds. Thinly slice one of the squeezed lemons, and place the slices on the fish. Finally, top with the onion slices.

2. Cook on Low for 3 to 4 hours or on High for 1 to 2 hours, until fish is cooked through and flakes easily.

Variation:

This simply prepared fish is also delicious chilled and served in lettuce wraps. Garnish with chopped cucumbers, cherry tomatoes, and a thin slice of avocado.

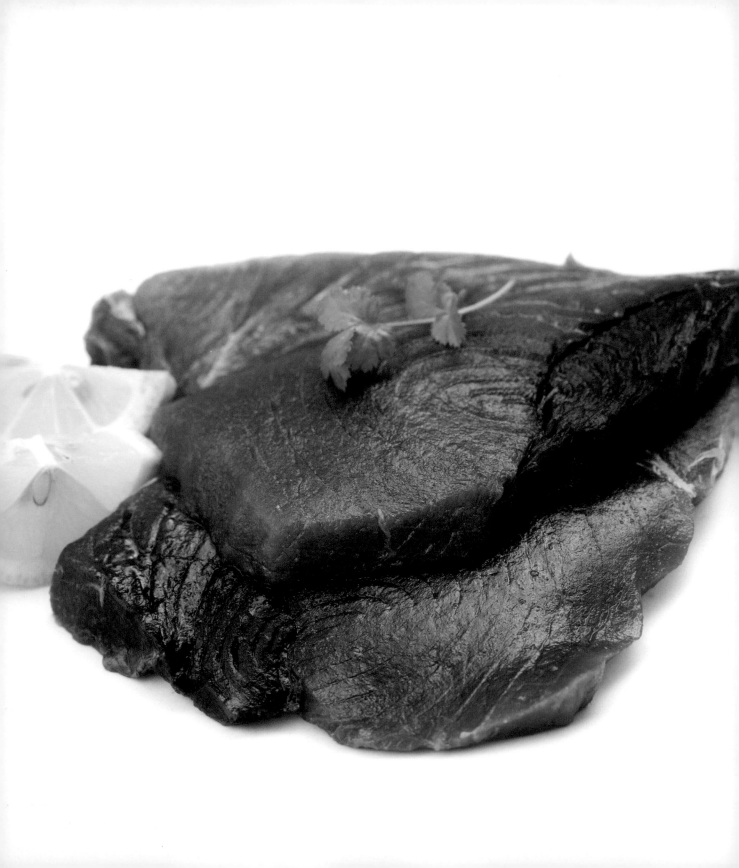

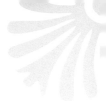

Tomato-Braised Tuna

Tuna is caught in the waters off Sicily, and in this recipe the gentle heat of the slow cooker glorifies this meaty fish while keeping it fairly rare. If you have any left over, you can add it to a mixed salad.

Makes 4 to 6 servings.

1½ to 2 pounds tuna fillet in one thick slice

¼ cup olive oil, divided

½ small red onion, chopped

3 cloves garlic, minced

15.5-oz can diced tomatoes

1 teaspoon fresh basil, chopped

¼ teaspoon dried oregano

½ teaspoon dried rosemary

3 tablespoons capers, drained and rinsed

2 tablespoons fresh parsley, chopped

1 bay leaf

Salt and pepper to taste

1. Soak tuna in cold water for 10 minutes. Pat dry with paper towels.

2. Heat 2 tablespoons of the oil in a large skillet over medium-high heat. Add onion and garlic and cook, stirring frequently, for 3 minutes, or until onion is translucent. Scrape mixture into the slow cooker. Add diced tomatoes, herbs, capers, parsley, and bay leaf to the slow cooker and stir well. Cook on Low for 2 to 3 hours or on High for about 1 hour.

3. Heat remaining oil in the skillet over medium-high heat. Add tuna, and brown well on both sides. Add tuna to the slow cooker, and cook on Low for an additional 2 hours or on High for an additional hour or 90 minutes. Tuna should be cooked but still rare in the center. Remove and discard bay leaf, season to taste with salt and pepper, and serve hot. Garnish with lemon wedges, if desired.

Soaking the tuna in water removes a lot of its remaining blood, so that the finished dish is lighter in color and not bright red. The same treatment can be used on other dark fish, such as mackerel or bluefish.

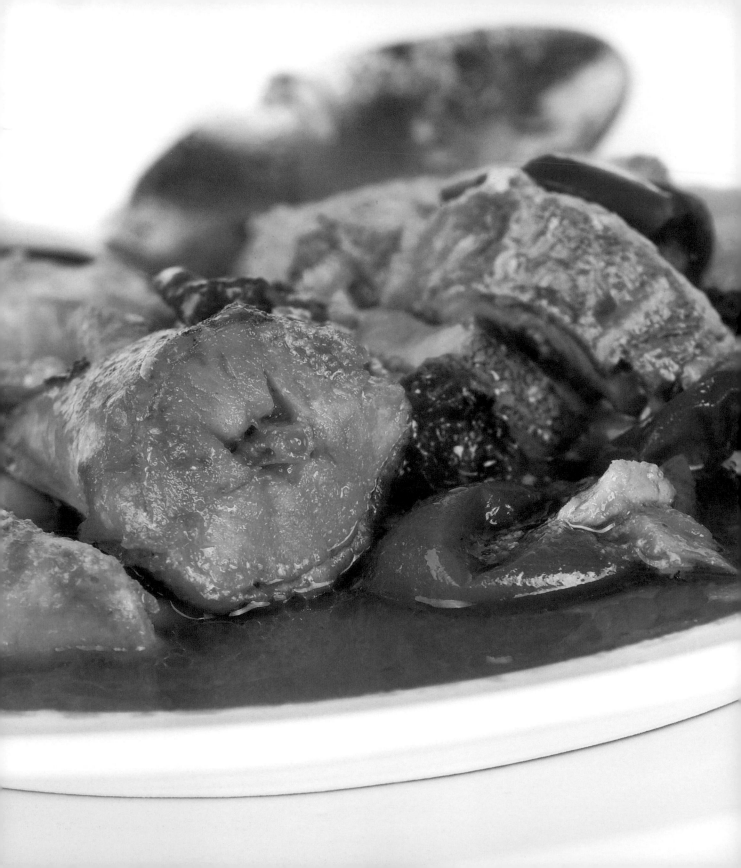

Fish Stew with Sausage

This stew is a hearty and flavorful dish, with both sausage and pancetta enlivening the flavor. Serve with a salad of tangy greens, like arugula.

Makes 4 to 6 servings.

½ pound thick cod fillet

½ pound swordfish fillet

½ pound bay scallops

2 juice oranges, washed

¼ pound pancetta or bacon, diced

1 medium onion, diced

1 carrot, sliced

1 celery rib, sliced

3 cloves garlic, minced

½ pound fresh pork sausage

14.5-oz can diced tomatoes, undrained

3½ cups fish stock or broth

3 tablespoons fresh basil, chopped

2 tablespoons fresh parsley, chopped

1 tablespoon fresh thyme, chopped

1 bay leaf

Salt and pepper to taste

1. Rinse fish and pat dry with paper towels. Remove and discard any skin or bones. Cut fish into 1-inch cubes. Refrigerate fish and scallops until ready to use, tightly covered with plastic wrap. Grate off zest, and then squeeze oranges for juice. Set aside.

2. Cook pancetta in a heavy skillet over medium-high heat for about 4 minutes, or until browned. Remove from the pan with a slotted spoon, and transfer the pancetta to the slow cooker. Discard all but 2 tablespoons of the grease.

3. Add onion, carrot, celery, garlic, and sausage to the skillet. Cook, stirring frequently, for about 3 minutes, or until onion is translucent. Scrape mixture into the slow cooker.

4. Add tomatoes, orange zest, orange juice, stock, basil, parsley, thyme, and bay leaf to the slow cooker, and stir well. Cook on Low for 6 to 8 hours or on High for 3 to 4 hours, until vegetables are soft.

5. If cooking on Low, raise the heat to High. Add fish, and cook for 30 to 50 minutes, or until fish is cooked through and flakes easily. Remove and discard bay leaf. Season with salt and pepper.

Whenever zest from a citrus fruit is being added to a dish, wash the fruit with mild soap and water before grating the zest off. Many citrus growers spray with pesticides, and the residue remains on the fruit. Also, some fruit is lightly waxed before shipment to make it more transportable.

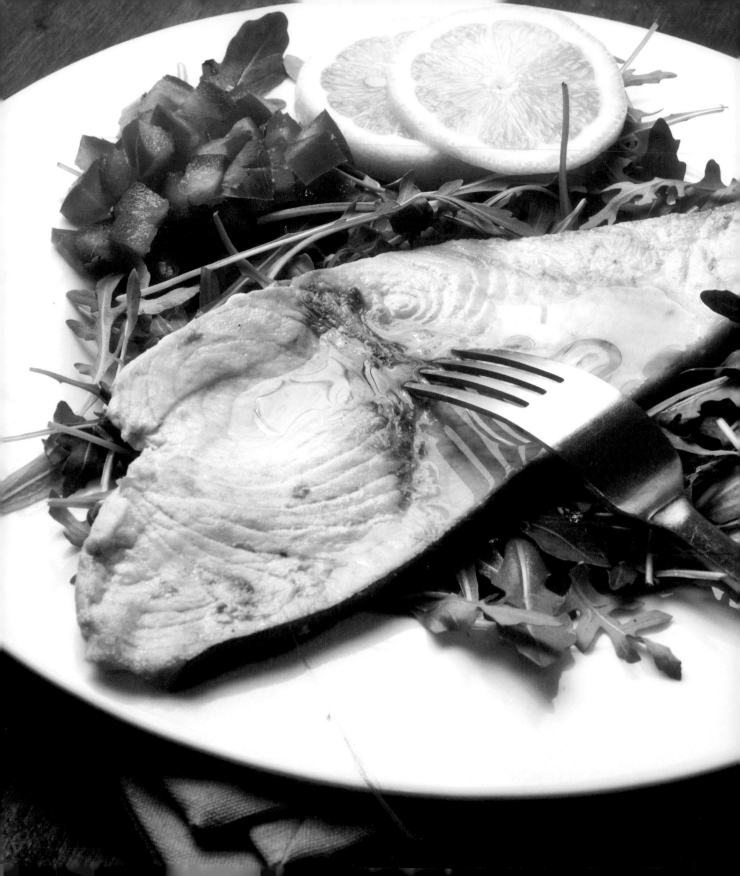

Swordfish with Lemon & Capers

Swordfish is such a wonderfully meaty fish that it stands up to some stronger seasonings, including capers. They add an extra tang to the lemony dish.

Makes 2 to 4 servings.

2 pounds swordfish steaks

Salt and pepper to taste

2 lemons

2 tablespoons capers

2 tablespoons clarified butter

¼ cup fish stock or water

1 tablespoon fresh dill, chopped

1. Put the swordfish steaks on a piece of aluminum foil that will be big enough to wrap over the fish to form a sealed cooking "tent." With the fish in the middle of the piece of foil, squeeze the juice of the lemons over them, removing seeds as you go. Sprinkle the fish with some salt and pepper, the put the capers over it. Cut the butter into small pieces and dot the steaks with it. Bring up the sides of the foil and begin to form the packet. When the sides are up, add the stock or water before securing all edges together and fully enclosing the fish.

2. Put the packet in the slow cooker. Cook on Low for 3 to 4 hours or on High for 2 to 3 hours. It's cooked when the flesh flakes easily but is still moist. Be careful not to overcook.

3. When serving, pour the sauce from the packet over the fish. Garnish with dill.

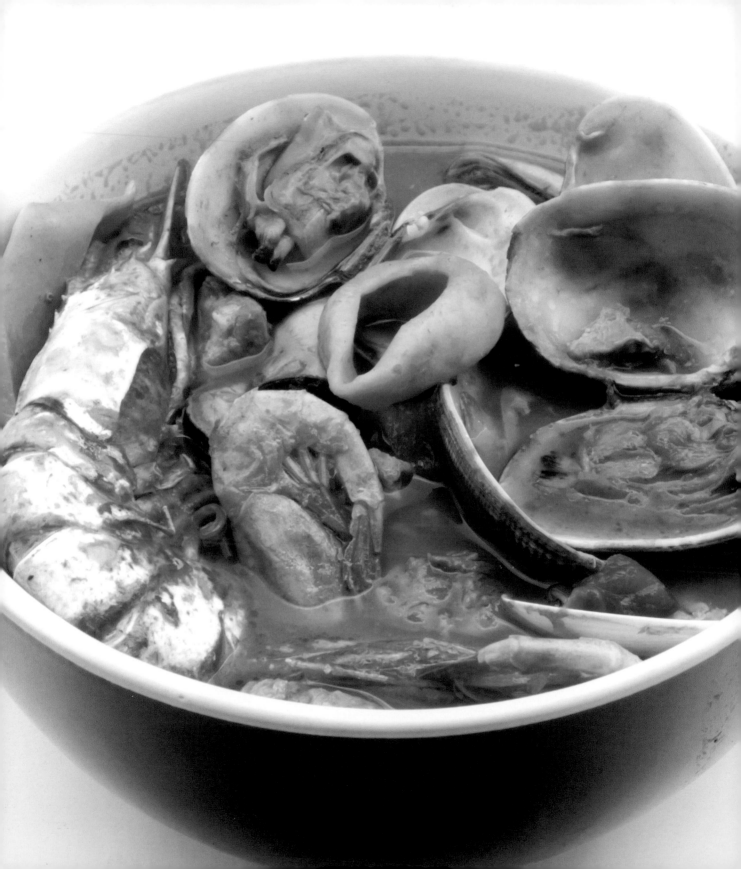

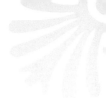

Pesce Magnifico

This amazing one-pot meal of assorted fish and shellfish is bursting with flavor with the freshness of herbs. It is an appropriate base for a wide range of fish, though you'll want to make sure it includes squid and shrimp.

Makes 4 to 6 servings.

1 large white onion, chopped

3 cloves garlic, minced

2 large stalks celery, fronds removed, finely chopped

1 red bell pepper, seeded and chopped

8 oz. clam juice

½ cup water

2 tablespoons extra virgin olive oil

1 tablespoon lemon zest

1 tablespoon fresh basil, chopped

1 tablespoon fresh parsley, chopped

1 teaspoon fresh oregano

1 teaspoon fresh thyme

1 bay leaf

1 pound thick, firm-fleshed white fish cut into 1 inch pieces

½ pound squid, cleaned and sliced

¾ pound shrimp, shelled and deveined

Salt to taste

¼ cup fresh parsley, chopped

1. In a large bowl, combine onions, garlic, celery, red pepper, clam juice, water, olive oil, zest, spices, and bay leaf. Mix well. Put into slow cooker

2. Cover and cook on Low for 4 to 5 hours or on High for 2 to 3 hours until vegetables are tender. If cooking on Low, increase heat to High. Remove and discard bay leaf. Add fish, squid, and shrimp and cook for an additional hour or so until fish is cooked through. Season with salt and pepper to taste, and garnish with fresh parsley.

Variations:

* Many fish that do beautifully in this recipe. Consider using tilapia, mackerel, sole, grouper, monk fish, whiting, or porgy (all boned, of course).

* Make it extra-Italian by adding chopped anchovies with the fish.

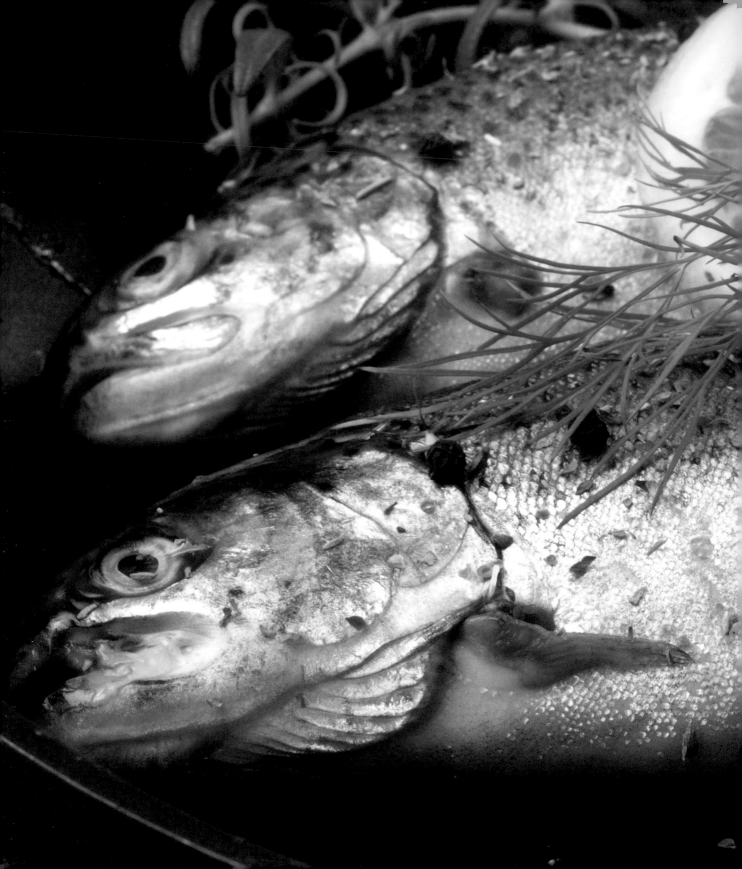

Brook Trout *Italiano*

The combination of oregano, basil, parsley, garlic, and rosemary make for a fragrant, delicious, and nutritious topping to this tender fish.

Makes 4 servings.

3 to 4 pounds brook trout fillets

¼ cup olive oil

2 cloves garlic, minced

1 teaspoon fresh oregano, chopped, or ¼ teaspoon dried

1 teaspoon fresh basil, chopped, or ½ teaspoon dried

1 teaspoon fresh parsley, chopped, or ½ teaspoon dried

1 teaspoon fresh rosemary, chopped, or ½ teaspoon dried

Juice of 1 lemon

¼ cup dry white wine

1. Place the fillets in the slow cooker. Add the garlic to the olive oil, and drizzle over the fish.

2. In a small bowl, combine the herbs and mix with a fork to blend without overly crushing. Sprinkle the herb mixture over the fish. Squeeze the lemon over the fish and add the wine.

3. Cook on Low for about 2 hours or on High for about 1 hour. The herbs will have made a thin carpet over the fish. Pour the juices from the cooker over the fish when serving. Season with salt and pepper.

It's easy to make your own Italian seasonings blend to have handy for seasoning fish, poultry, sauces, and even sprinkling on salads. Using dried herbs, combine 1 tablespoon each of the oregano, basil, parsley, and rosemary. Substitute 2 teaspoons garlic powder for the fresh garlic. Store in a small glass jar with an airtight lid.

Brook Trout with Lemon

This recipe calls for cooking the fish whole, but don't worry—filleting it when it's cooked is easy. It makes an elegant presentation on the plate, and there's something very satisfying about removing the skeleton yourself.

Makes 2 to 4 servings.

2 medium to large whole brook trout, cleaned by the fishmonger but not filleted

2 lemons

2 teaspoons herbes de Provence

Salt to taste

2 tablespoons clarified butter

⅔ cup dry white wine

1 tablespoon fresh parsley, chopped

1. Put 1 trout each on pieces of aluminum foil that are big enough to wrap over the fish to form a sealed cooking "tent." With the trout in the middle of the piece of foil, squeeze the juice of 1 lemon over each, removing seeds as you go. Sprinkle each fish with a teaspoon of herbes de Provence and some salt. Cut the butter into 4 small pieces and place two pats each on top of the fish. If desired, slice the lemons and place 2 slices in the cavity inside each fish.

2. Bring up the sides of the foil and begin to form the packet. When the sides are up, pour ⅓ cup wine on each trout before securing all edges together and fully enclosing the fish.

3. Put the trout packets in the slow cooker. Cook on Low for 2 to 3 hours or on High for 1 to 2 hours. Half way through, peek into one of the packets to see how the fish is doing. It's cooked when the flesh is pale and easily flakes away from the bones. Make sure it's cooked through before removing from packets and serving. Serve whole, pouring the sauce in the packet over the fish. Garnish with parsley.

Removing the trout's skeleton so your fish is free of bones is easy if you take your time. With the fish on your plate, loosen the flesh close to the spine and gently scrape/slide the top "fillet" off the skeleton. When it's off and half the skeleton is exposed, lift the head or tail of the trout and gently pull back and lift up to pull the remaining skeleton away from the fillet on the bottom. Discard the skeleton.

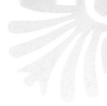

Monkfish Kebobs

The nice thing about making kabobs in the slow cooker is that you don't have to worry about parts or all of them burning on the grill.

Makes 4 to 6 servings.

⅓ cup olive oil

1 tablespoon Italian seasoning

2 cloves garlic, mashed

¼ teaspoon salt

½ teaspoon pepper

2 pounds salmon, cut into cubes

1 red bell pepper, seeded and cut into large chunks

1 green bell pepper, seeded and cut into large chunks

1 onion, cut into thick wedges

2 quarts ripe cherry tomatoes

1 zucchini, cut into thin slices

Wooden skewers, cut or broken into sizes to fit into the slow cooker

1. In a large bowl, combine the olive oil, herbs, garlic, salt and pepper, and stir to combine. Add the fish, peppers, onions, and zucchini, and toss to coat all.

2. Put the fish and vegetables onto the skewers, working in the cherry tomatoes. Put the skewers in the slow cooker as you finish them. Pour the remaining dressing over the skewers.

3. Cook on Low for 3 to 4 hours or on High for 2 to 3 hours until fish is cooked through and vegetables are crisp-tender.

Variation:

Turn up the Italian in this recipe by adding fresh basil. You can either put whole leaves on the skewers as you make them, or shred some leaves to yield ½ cup and sprinkle them over the cooked kebabs.

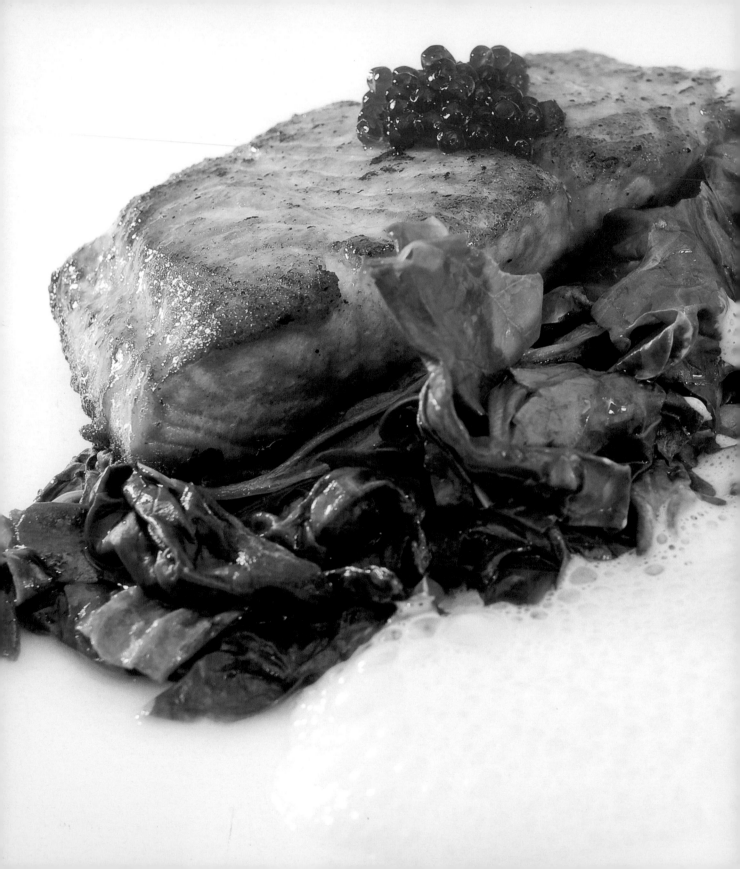

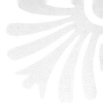

Salmon with Spinach

This is a great throw-together meal for busy households because you can use frozen salmon fillets. Thaw them by placing each fillet in an air-tight plastic baggie and submersing in a bowl of cool water. It takes about 20 minutes to thaw several fillets at once.

Makes 2 to 4 servings.

4 frozen salmon fillets, thawed

Four 16-oz bags fresh baby spinach greens (or a spinach/kale combo)

2 cloves garlic, minced

2 tablespoons coconut oil

Salt to taste

2 tablespoons toasted sesame seeds

1. Working in batches, put spinach in the colander and give it a quick rinse, picking through the leaves and removing any large stems. Shake excess water from the spinach, but don't dry thoroughly. Put spinach in slow cooker after rinsing. When all spinach is in the slow cooker, add the garlic and oil and stir to combine and coat the leaves.

2. Place the salmon fillets on top of the spinach greens. Cook on Low for about 1 hour, until spinach is wilted and fish is cooked through. Depending on how well done you like your salmon, you may want to cook it an additional 15 to 20 minutes.

3. In a small, dry skillet over medium-high heat, add the sesame seeds and cook, shaking lightly or stirring to keep the seeds from sticking and burning, until seeds are lightly toasted, about 2 minutes. Garnish salmon and spinach with the sesame seeds, and season with salt to taste.

One of the reasons for eliminating grain is that it is the cause of inflammation. Frozen fish fillets are usually from farm-raised fish that are grown in pens and often fed with grains. For this reason, people looking to get the most out of their Paleo diet should choose wild-caught over farm-raised fish.

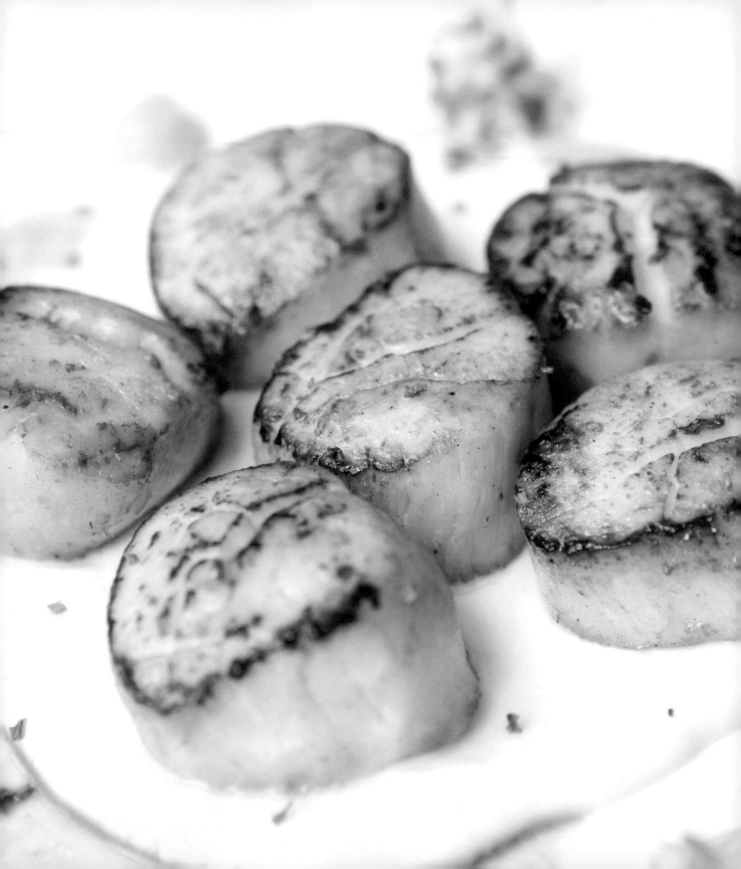

Scallops with *Noce* (Walnuts)

Scallops are a very meaty fish, which is just what you want for this recipe. Its delicate taste but firm texture holds up well to the earthy walnut sauce that accompanies it.

Makes 4 to 6 servings.

3 pounds medium-sized scallops

Salt and pepper

1 cup dry white wine

½ cup olive oil

1 small onion, chopped

2 cloves garlic, sliced thin

½ cup walnut pieces, lightly toasted

½ cup fresh-squeezed lemon juice, seeds removed

½ cup water

1 tablespoon coconut oil

1 tablespoon fresh parsley, chopped

1. Rinse scallops and pat dry. Season lightly with salt and pepper. Put the wine in the slow cooker and add the scallops. Cover and cook on Low for 3 to 4 hours or on High for 60 to 90 minutes.

2. While scallops are cooking, prepare the walnut sauce. In a skillet, cook the onion and garlic in the olive oil over medium heat until the onion is translucent, about 3 minutes. Reduce the heat and add the walnuts. Continue to cook, stirring, for about 5 minutes. Transfer the mix to a food processor.

3. Working slowly at first, pulse the mix into a chunky paste. Add the lemon juice and pulse some more. Slowly stream in water and pulse to form a thick sauce. Scoop into a bowl and season with salt and pepper.

4. When scallops are cooked (firm throughout), heat the coconut oil in a large skillet on high heat. Scoop the scallops into the pan and flash-sear for about 2 minutes per side. Spread the walnut sauce on a platter and serve the scallops on top. Sprinkle with chopped parsley.

Selecting fresh scallops can be confusing. There are bay scallops, sea scallops, jumbo scallops, king scallops, cape scallops, and more! The easiest thing to remember is that bay scallops are small, and sea scallops are big. Another thing to look for is how the scallops are presented. Often they're packed in a phosphate solution to whiten and keep them plump. Avoid scallops treated that way by asking for "dry" scallops or chemical-free scallops.

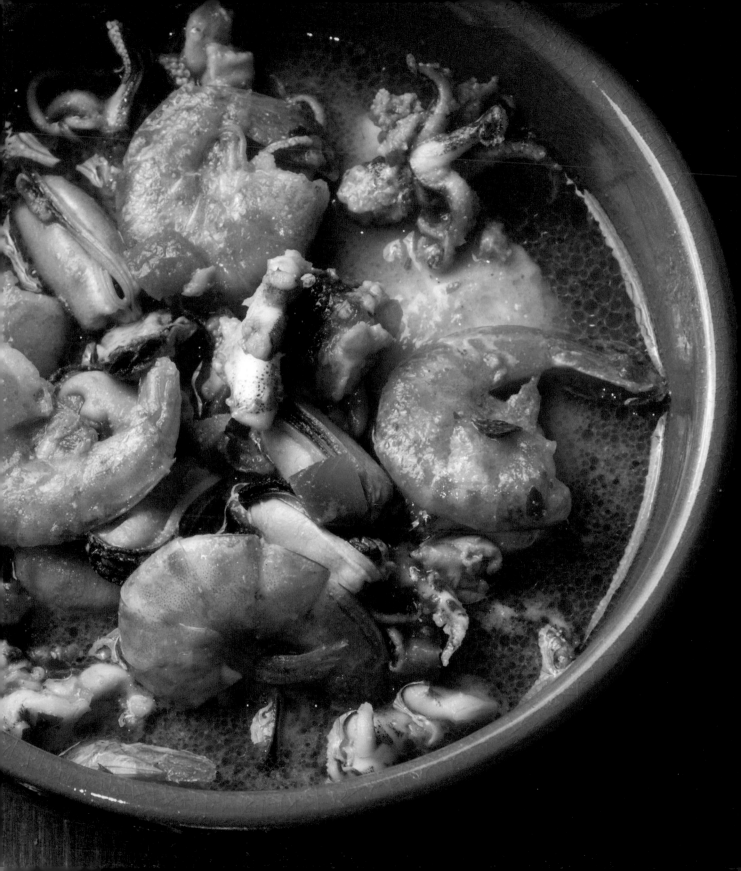

Hearty Shellfish Stew

This is the sort of fish stew that has become known as Cioppino in San Francisco and other American cities.

Makes 4 to 6 servings.

¾ pound thick firm-fleshed fish fillets, such as cod, swordfish, or halibut

¾ pound sea scallops

¼ pound extra-large shrimp

1 dozen mussels, scrubbed and debearded

3 tablespoons coconut oil

2 medium onions, diced

1 red bell pepper, seeds and ribs removed, and finely chopped

2 celery ribs, diced

3 cloves garlic, minced

2 tablespoons fresh oregano, chopped

2 teaspoons fresh thyme

28-oz can diced tomatoes, undrained

1½ cups dry red wine

2 tablespoons tomato paste

1 cup fish stock

1 bay leaf

¼ cup fresh parsley, chopped

3 tablespoons fresh basil, chopped

Salt and pepper to taste

1. Rinse fish and pat dry with paper towels. Remove and discard any skin of bones. Cut fish into 1-inch cubes.

2. Cut scallops in half. Peel and devein the shrimp. Refrigerate all seafood until ready to use, tightly covered with plastic wrap.

3. Heat oil in a medium skillet over medium-high heat. Add onions, red bell pepper, celery, garlic, oregano, and thyme. Cook stirring frequently, for 3 minutes, or until onions are translucent. Scrape mixture into the slow cooker.

4. Add tomatoes, stock, tomato paste, and bay leaf to the slow cooker and stir well to dissolve tomato paste. Cook on Low for 5 to 7 hours or on High for 2 to 3 hours, until vegetables are almost tender.

5. If cooking on Low, raise the heat to High. Add seafood, parsley, and basil. Cook for 30 to 45 minutes, or until fish is cooked through. Remove and discard bay leaf, and season to taste with salt and pepper.

Variation:
Substitute squid for the sea scallops. Clean them, slice the bodies into ½-inch rings, and keep the tentacles whole.

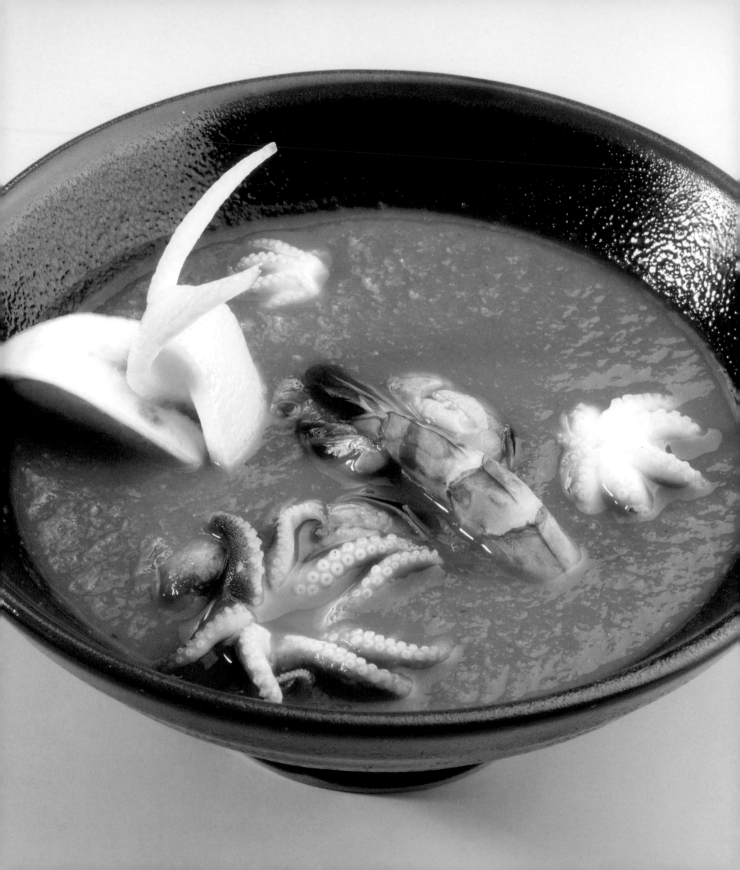

Octopus and Shrimp Soup

This is a soup in a chapter for main dishes, but I couldn't resist. It's a seafood lover's bonanza, just like the shellfish stew or bouillabase. Enjoy!

Makes 6 to 8 servings.

4 cups water

4 cups fish stock or broth

2 pounds octopus, cut into 1 inch pieces

1 tablespoon coconut oil

2 cups diced carrots

1 cup diced celery

½ cup chopped onion

14.5-ounce can diced tomatoes, drained

1 teaspoon crushed red pepper flakes (optional)

1½ pounds large shrimp (in shells)

Salt and pepper

1. In a skillet over medium heat, warm the coconut oil. Add the carrots, celery, and onion and cook, stirring, for about 5 minutes. Add the tomatoes and pepper flakes (if desired). Transfer the vegetable mix to the slow cooker.

2. Combine the water and fish stock and pour into the slow cooker. Add the octopus pieces. Cover and cook on Low for 8 to 10 hours or on High for 5 to 7 hours.

3. The octopus pieces should be tender and the broth hot. Turn the heat to High and shrimp in their shells. Cover and cook on High for about 1 hour, until the shrimp are cooked through. Season with salt and pepper. Scoop into large bowls.

Octopus is typically sold frozen. This is a good thing, as it spoils quickly when caught. Also, frozen octopus is usually cleaned before being frozen, which means the home cook doesn't have to worry about which parts to cut off before using. Thaw the fish at room temperature until ready to use.

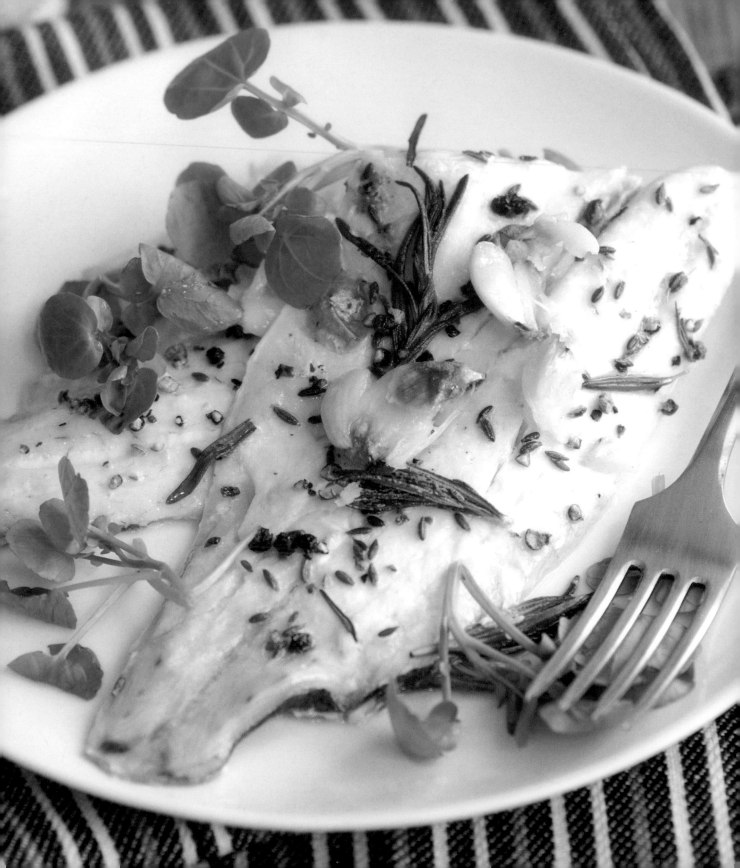

Lemon-Thyme Sea Bass

Sea bass is a delicately flavored fish, and you don't need a lot of thyme to give it a nice flavor without overwhelming it. Leeks have a milder flavor than onions, too, and work well in this dish. You could give it a hint of heat by sprinkling with paprika.

Makes 4 to 6 servings.

3 pounds sea bass fillet

1 tablespoon fresh thyme, chopped

2 lemons

2 leeks, white part only, thinly sliced and thoroughly washed

Salt and pepper to taste

1. Make sure the fillets are free of bones. Put them skin side down into the slow cooker. Sprinkle the thyme over the fish, then squeeze the lemons over them. Remove any seeds. Thinly slice one of the squeezed lemons, and place the slices on the fish. Finally, top with the leek slices.

2. Cook on Low for 3 to 4 hours or on High for 1 to 2 hours, until fish is cooked through and flakes easily.

The sea bass is a relative of the grouper. The fish available in American markets is black sea bass, which are fished off of the Atlantic Coast. At one time their populations were dwindling, and restrictions were put on how many fish could be caught. The populations have resurged, but are still threatened, and restrictions remain in place. So when it's available, take advantage!

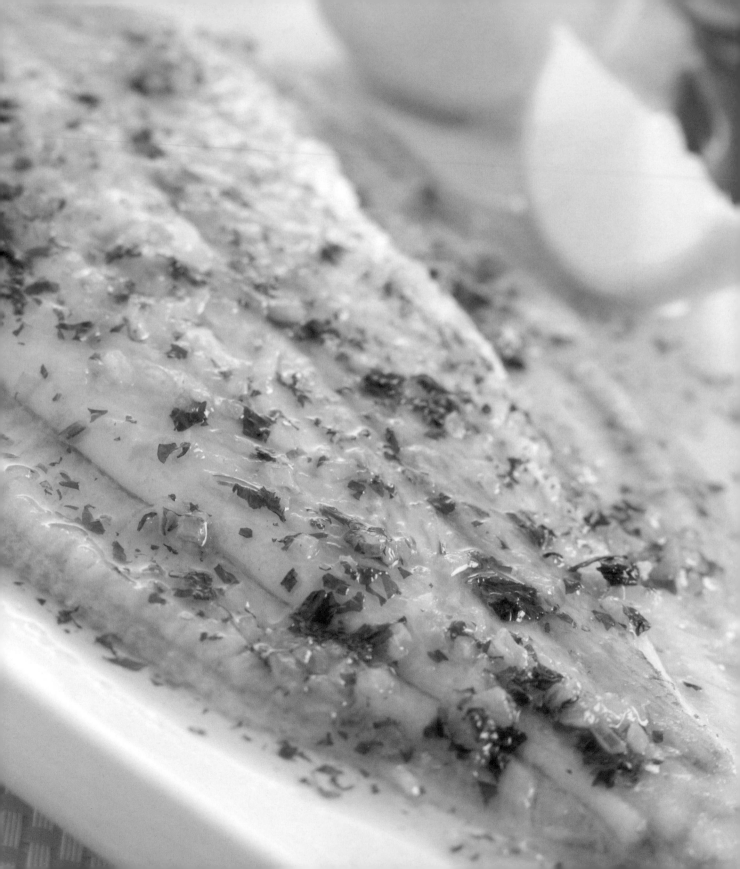

Poached Sole

A foil packet tucked inside your slow cooker is a great way to prepare a simple fish dish, in much the same way you'd do it on the grill or in the oven.

Makes 4 to 6 servings.

2 pounds sole

2 tablespoons olive oil

1 tablespoon fresh-squeezed lemon juice

4 sprigs fresh herbs

4 thin slices lemon

Salt and pepper

Heavy-duty aluminum foil

1. Place an oversized piece of heavy-duty aluminum foil in the slow cooker. Put the fish on the foil. Season with salt and pepper. Drizzle with olive oil and lemon juice. Top with the herbs and lemon slices.

2. Using another piece of foil, cover the fish and tightly wrap every edge of the foil to create a sealed foil packet. Cover and cook on Low for 3 to 5 hours or on High for 1 to 2 hours. When you open the foil packet, the fish will be poached in a lemon-herb sauce. Serve immediately.

Sole is a relative of the flounder. Wild-caught sole comes from the Pacific Ocean. When shopping for this fish, check whether it's farm-raised or fresh-caught, and ask about its origin. Being a delicate fish, you want something with maximum flavor and freshness.

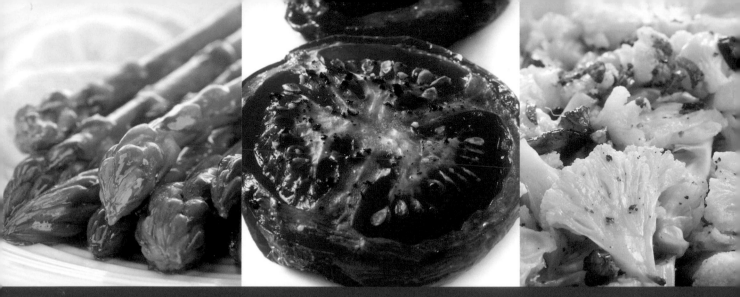

Chapter 8

Paleo Contorni:

Vegetables and Sides

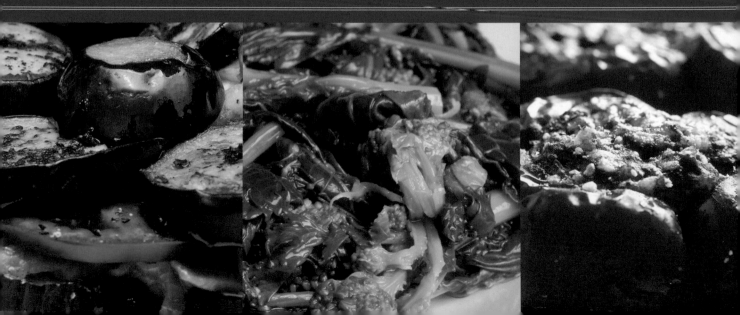

The gardens of Italy have been yielding amazing vegetables for millennia. Earthy mushrooms, broccoli, eggplant, and artichokes. Peppers of all colors. Root vegetables like beets, Brussels sprouts, leeks, and squash. Tender asparagus. All are delicious when slow cooked in combination with other vegetables or with some additional meat or even eggs. And of course, garlic! There is no limit to the amount of color and flavor you can concoct as *contorni magnifico* for you, your family, and your guests.

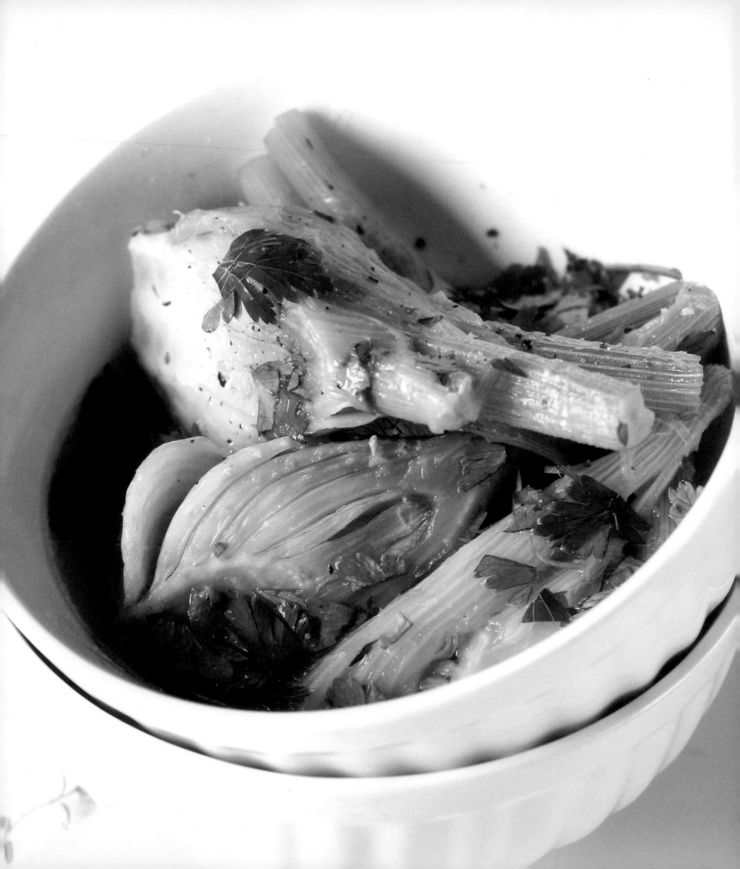

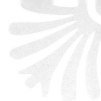

Braised Fennel

Fennel has an almost silky texture and sweet flavor once it's braised, and this dish goes with almost anything and everything, especially dishes with dark colors and assertive seasonings.

Makes 4 to 6 servings.

2 medium fennel bulbs, about 1 pound each

2 tablespoons coconut butter

½ small onion, thinly sliced

1 clove garlic, minced

1 cup vegetable stock or broth

1 teaspoon fresh thyme, or ¼ teaspoon dried

Salt and pepper to taste

1. Cut stalks off fennel bulb, trim root end, and cut bulb in half through the root. Trim out core, then slice fennel into 1-inch-thick slices across the bulb. Arrange slices in the slow cooker, and repeat with second bulb.

2. Heat butter in a small skillet over medium heat. Add onion and garlic and cook, stirring frequently, for 3 minutes, or until onion is translucent. Scrape mixture into the slow cooker.

3. Add stock and thyme to the slow cooker. Cook on Low for 4 to 6 hours or on High for 2 to 3 hours, or until fennel is tender. Season to taste with salt and pepper.

Although the celery-like stalks are trimmed off the fennel bulb for this dish, don't throw them out. They add a wonderful anise flavor as well as a crisp texture and are used in place of celery in salads and other raw dishes.

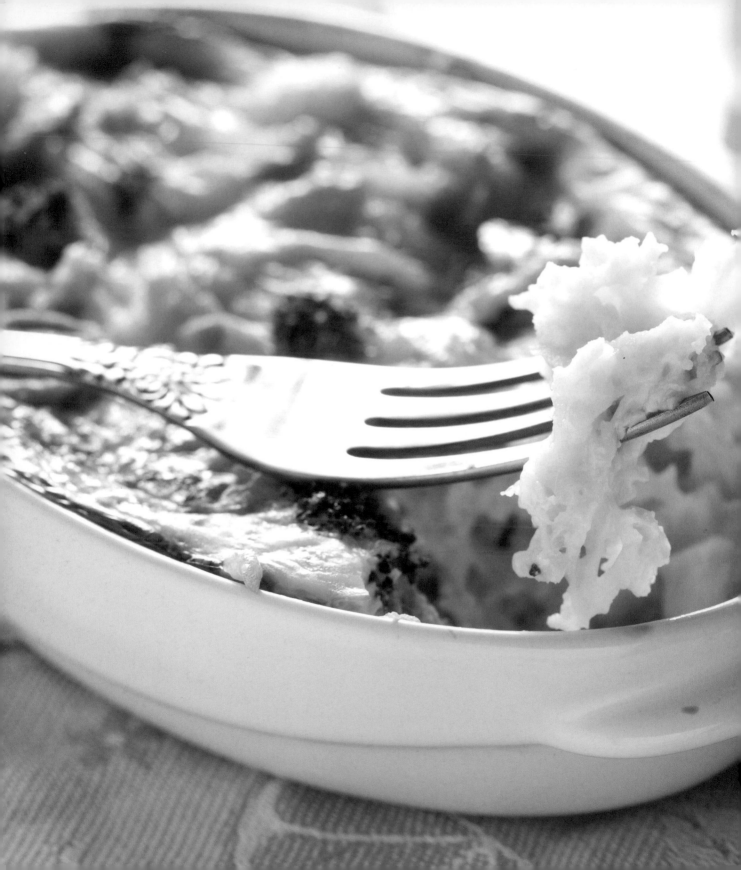

Fritatta con Cavofiliore

The southern part of Italy has many Arab influences, as North Africa is but a sliver of ocean away. This delicious frittata recipe with cauliflower and fresh parsley also contains the spice harissa, which adds a delicious zing!

Makes 4 to 6 servings.

2 tablespoons olive oil

1 small onion, finely chopped

2 garlic cloves, minced

¼ pound thick-sliced bacon, cut into 1-inch pieces

½ head cauliflower

8 eggs

Salt and freshly ground pepper to taste

½ cup fresh parsley, chopped fine, plus some for garnish

2 teaspoons ground caraway seeds

½ teaspoon harissa dissolved in 1 teaspoon water (or ¼ tsp cayenne)

Freshly ground pepper

1. Heat the oil in a heavy skillet over medium heat and add the onion. Cook, stirring, until the onion is just translucent, about 3 minutes. Add the garlic and stir together for another minute or so. Transfer the mixture to the slow cooker.

2. In the still-hot skillet, cook the bacon pieces until crispy. Remove the pan from the heat and scoop out the bacon pieces with a slotted spoon so that the fat stays in the pan. Put the bacon in the slow cooker.

3. Trim the cauliflower of any leaves and remove the coarse bottom of the stem. Chop the rest into large chunks and medium-sized florets. Steam the cauliflower in a pot of boiling salted water for about 15 minutes, until tender. Drain. Put the cooked cauliflower in a bowl, and mash it with a fork until it is crumbly. Add to the onion/garlic mixture in the slow cooker.

4. In a large bowl, whisk the eggs and season with salt and freshly ground pepper. Add the parsley and caraway seeds, then the harissa or cayenne. Stir, and pour over the other ingredients in the slow cooker. Stir gently to combine. Cook on Low for 6 to 8 hours or on High for 3 to 4 hours until set. Garnish with fresh parsley. Serve at room temperature.

Harissa is a seasoning paste or sauce made from roasted peppers including red bell, Serrano, and hot chili peppers. It also contains garlic, chili powder, coriander and caraway seeds. Originating in Tunisia, it is used widely in North Africa as a seasoning for couscous and meat dishes and is also commonly available in Italy, France, and Germany.

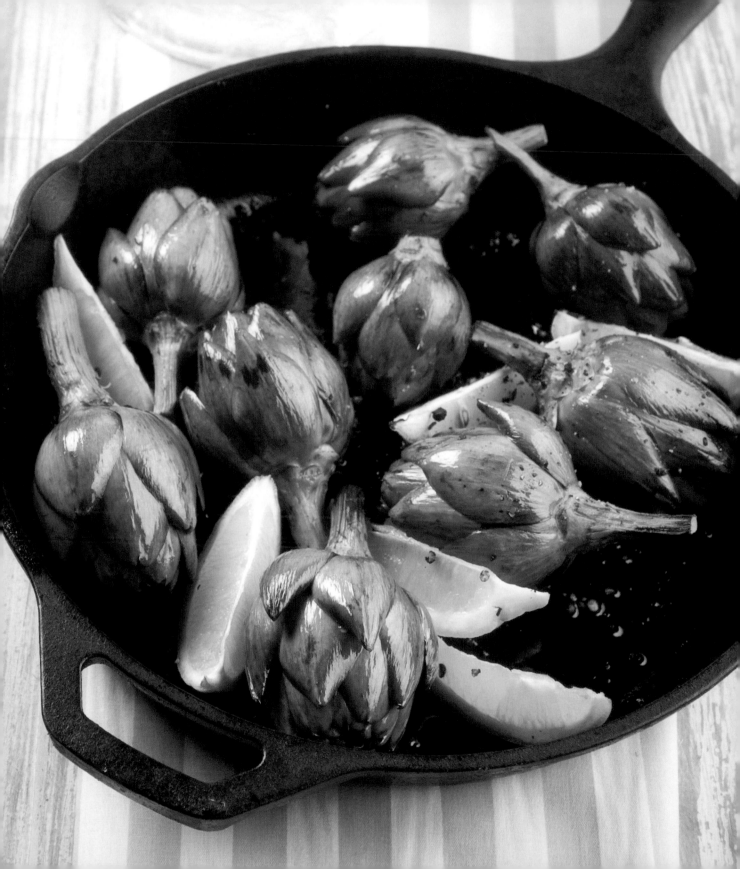

Artichokes with Lemon & Herbs

Don't be intimidated by their prickly exterior. Artichokes are easily prepared in the slow cooker.

Makes 4 to 6 servings.

4 to 6 artichokes, depending on size of vegetables and the slow cooker

1 lemon, quartered

3 cloves garlic, crushed

1 teaspoon fresh rosemary, minced

2 cups water

1. Wash and pat dry the artichokes. Trim the stem to about ¼ inch from bottom. Pull off the first couple of layers of leaves at the bottom, and snip the pointy ends off the leaves all around the chokes.

2. Place the artichokes in the slow cooker, bottoms down. Squeeze the juice of the lemons over the artichokes and put the squeezed quarters in with the artichokes, distributed throughout. Peel the garlic cloves and crush with the back of a knife. Put the garlic cloves in the slow cooker, distributed throughout. Sprinkle the rosemary around the artichokes.

3. Pour the water around the artichokes so that it covers the bottom of the slow cooker with about ½ to 1 inch of water. Cover and cook on Low for 6 to 8 hours or on High for 4 to 5 hours. Artichokes should be tender, with leaves easily breaking away from the core. Serve hot or at room temperature with the lemon/garlic juice as a dipping sauce for the leaves.

Artichokes are a lot of fun to eat as you work your way through the leaves to what is considered the vegetable's most delicious part, its heart. Peel each leaf off and dip the bottom into the lemon/garlic cooking liquid, or into some melted coconut butter. Put the leaf in your mouth, press down with your teeth, and scrape the tender flesh from the lower part of the leaves. Work through the artichoke until the leaves are small and nearly transparent. Pull off the last tip of leaves. The heart will be left, attached to the stem. There is some "fuzz" on the top of the heart that needs to be gently scraped off, as it can be bitter. It falls off easily. Now enjoy the heart!

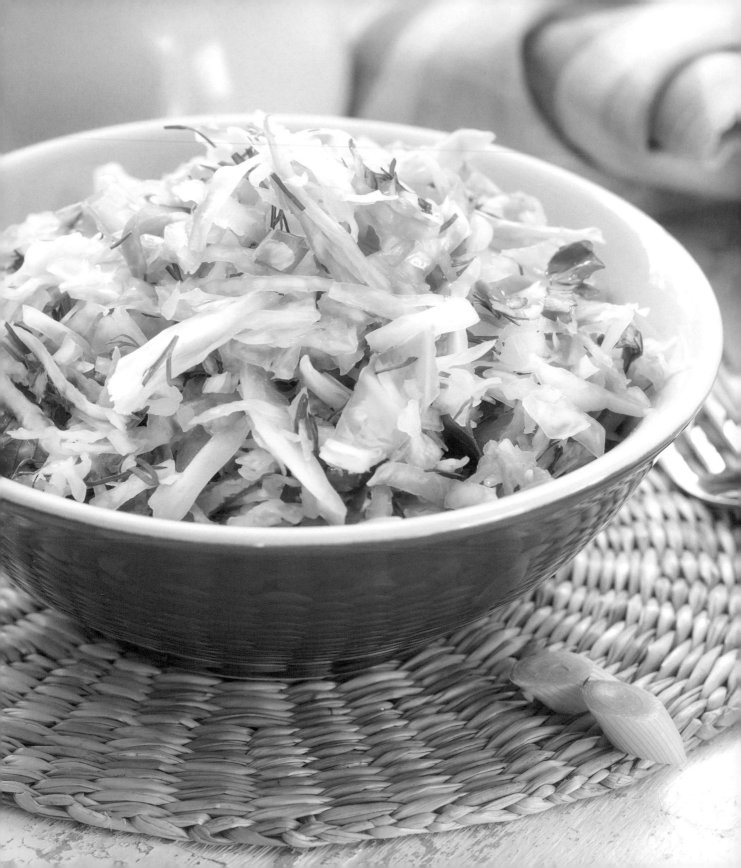

Sardinian-Style Cabbage

This cabbage dish is subtly flavored with pancetta and herbs, and the braising makes it a tender treat for any winter meal.

Makes 6 to 8 servings.

2 tablespoons olive oil

¼ pound pancetta, diced

2 cloves garlic, minced

1 large head (1½ pounds) green cabbage, shredded

2 tablespoons fresh chopped parsley

1 bay leaf

1 cup chicken stock or broth

Salt and pepper to taste

1. Heat oil in a large skillet over medium-high heat. Add pancetta, stirring frequently, and cook for 4 to 5 minutes, or until browned. Add garlic, and cook for 30 seconds, stirring constantly. Add cabbage, parsley, bay leaf, and stock, and bring to a boil. Scrape mixture into the slow cooker.

2. Cook on Low for 5 to 7 hours or on High for 2 to 3 hours, or until cabbage softens. Remove and discard bay leaf, season to taste with salt and pepper.

An advantage of cooking cruciferous vegetables such as cabbage, cauliflower or broccoli in the slow cooker is that the house doesn't smell like vegetables for days, which many people find offensive. This is because very little liquid evaporates from the slow cooker, and it's the steam in the air that carries the fragrance.

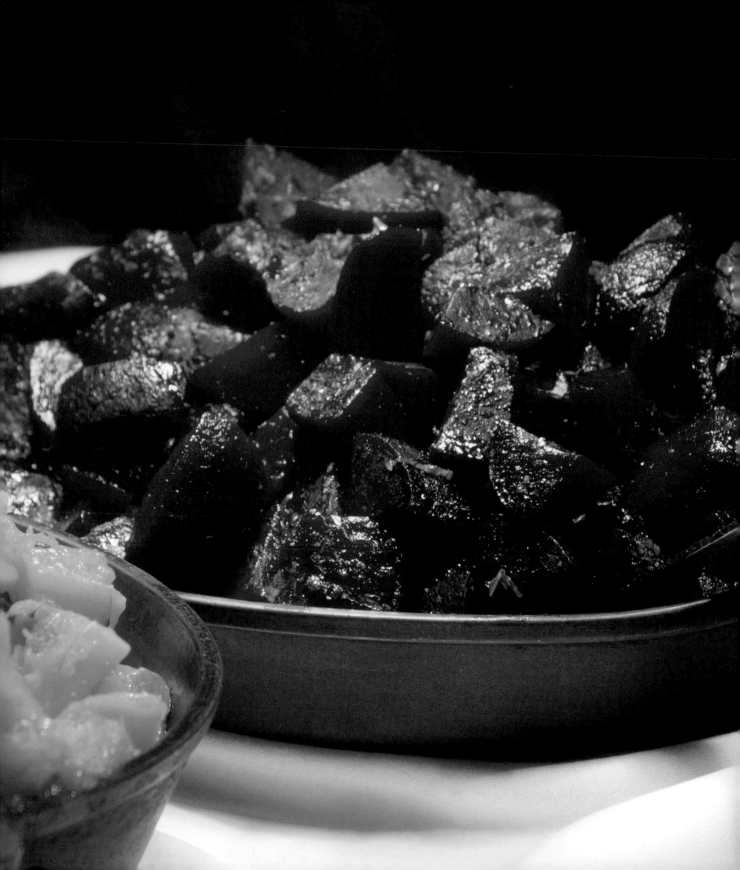

Slow-Roasted Beets

If you love beets, you'll love this method of cooking them. It "beats" waiting a long time for them to cook in boiling water!

Makes 6 to 8 servings.

2 bunches beets with tops (about 2 pounds)

2 tablespoons olive oil

1 clove garlic, minced

Greens from the beets, washed and cut into 1-inch pieces

Salt to taste

1. Scrub the beets clean and cut into 1-inch pieces.

2. Heat the oil in a medium skillet over medium-high heat and add the garlic. Cook, stirring constantly, about 1 minute. Add the beet greens and continue cooking and stirring until greens are just wilted, about 3 minutes.

3. Put beets into the slow cooker, topping with the greens. Cover and cook on low for 4 to 5 hours, or on high for 3 to 4 hours, or until beets are soft. Season with salt and serve.

Betacynin is the name of the pigment that gives red beets their deep color. Some people's bodies aren't able to process betacynin during digestion. As a result, their urine may be colored pink. This is temporary and is in no way harmful.

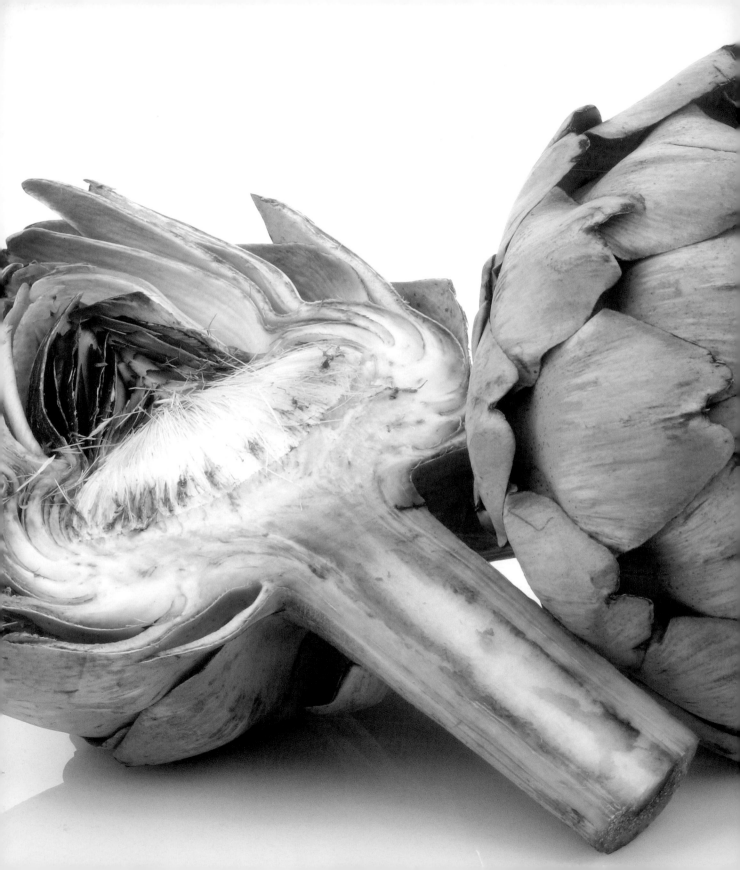

Braised Artichokes

Quartering the artichokes decreases the cooking time while still yielding the delicious slow-cooked goodness of the whole choke. The quarters are tender enough to eat whole, without having to peel off the leaves to eat the fleshy parts.

Makes 4 to 6 servings.

2 to 3 large artichokes
2 tablespoons coconut butter
2 cloves garlic, minced
1½ cups vegetable stock or broth
1 lemon, juiced
1 tablespoon fresh parsley, chopped
Salt and pepper to taste

1. Wash and pat dry the artichokes. Trim the stems back, snip off the pointy ends of the leaves, and cut into quarters. Arrange sections in the slow cooker.

2. Heat butter in a small skillet over medium heat and in it cook the garlic until just soft and perfumed, about 2 minutes. Scrape butter and garlic mixture into the slow cooker.

3. Add stock so that it is about ½- to 1-inch deep in the cooker. It should nearly cover the sections. Cover and cook on Low for 4 to 6 hours or on High for 2 to 3 hours, until artichoke sections are tender throughout. Add parsley and cook on low for another 10 to 15 minutes. Season to taste with salt and pepper.

The artichokes found in the United States are grown in California, though it was Mediterranean European countries where the vegetables originated and have been eaten for centuries. The name comes from the Italian word *articoclos*, which is said to refer to a pine cone. It is part of the thistle family, and plants grow three to six feet tall. The vegetable is the plant's flower bud, harvested before it flowers.

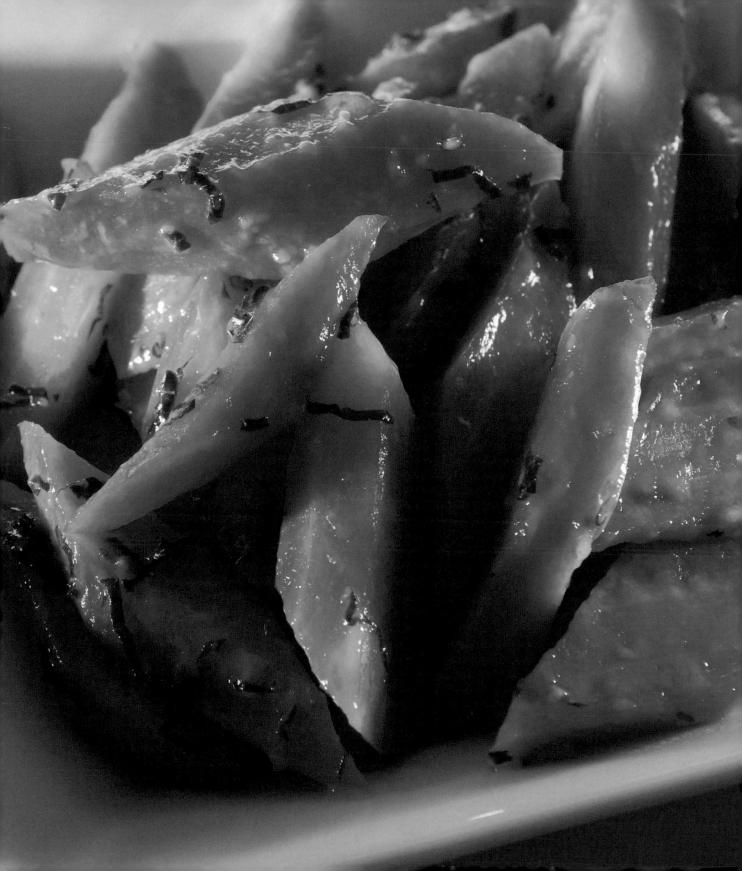

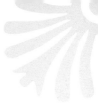

Herb-Seasoned Carrots

Adding a hint of something sweet to slow-cooked carrots turns them from tasty to terrific.

Makes 4 to 6 servings.

2 pounds carrots, peeled and cut quartered lengthwise into 4-inch sticks

½ cup vegetable broth or water

1 tablespoon coconut crystals or maple syrup

1 teaspoon olive oil

2 tablespoons fresh parsley or dill, chopped

1. Place carrot sticks in slow cooker. In a small bowl, combine the broth or water, coconut crystals or syrup, and olive oil. Pour the liquid over the carrots.

2. Cover and cook on Low for 2 hours until carrots are tender. Open the lid and keep it propped open with the handle of a wooden spoon, and continue to cook for 20 to 30 minutes until some liquid is cooked off and the carrots glaze. Garnish with fresh parsley or dill before serving.

> Carrots could be considered Paleo "candy"—a vegetable that also has a fairly high sugar content. Fortunately that sugar is naturally occurring and a "treat" in the truest sense of the word. Carrots are loaded with other vitamins and minerals, most notably beta carotene, from which they get their color. The brighter the better!

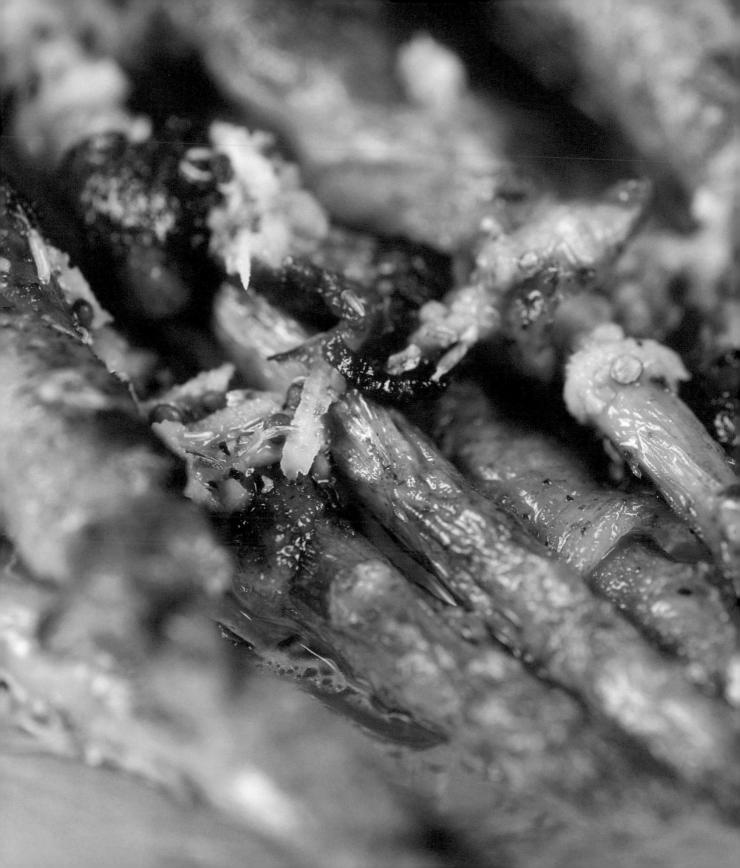

Asparagus with Pancetta

These wrapped asparagus are delicious, of course, but also make great snacks. They're fun to eat.

Makes 6 to 8 servings.

1 pound asparagus

1 pound pancetta, sliced very thin

1 tablespoon clarified butter or ghee, melted

1. Wash and dry asparagus spears, trimming off tough bottoms by about an inch.

2. Wrap each spear in a slice of pancetta, and lay the spears gently and carefully in the slow cooker.

3. Drizzle the spears with the melted butter. Cover and cook on Low for about 2 hours or on High for about 1 hour, until spears are tender.

4. Turn heat to high and cook for an additional 15 to 20 minutes with the lid propped open with the handle of a wooden spoon to allow steam to escape. This will dry-crisp the pancetta somewhat.

While thin spears are usually more desirable for quick cooking when steaming asparagus, for this recipe it is preferable to select fatter spears so there is more inside the wrap of pancetta.

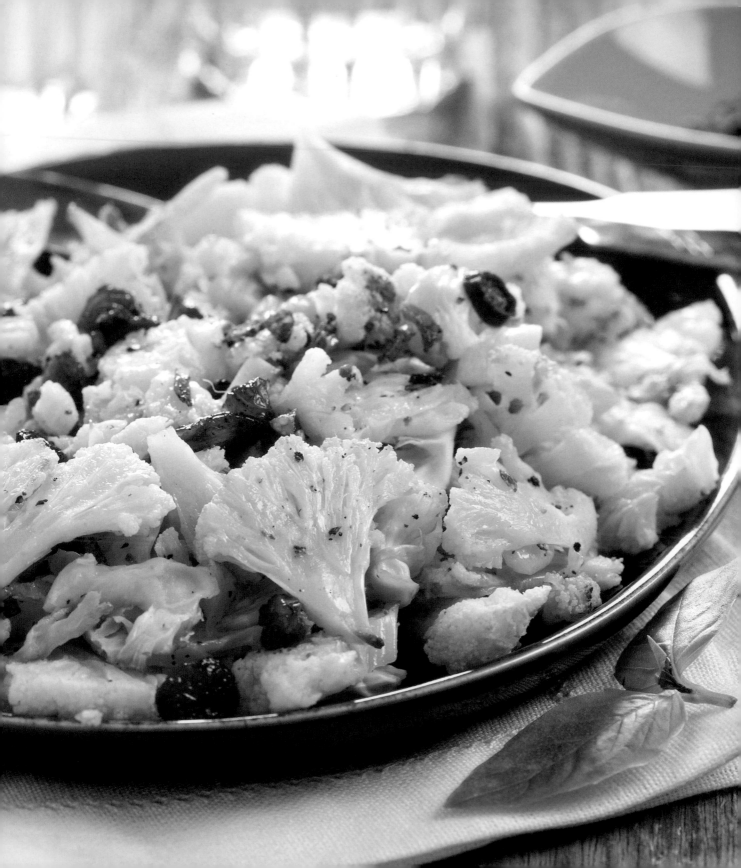

Cauliflower with Raisins and Pine Nuts

In Italy this dish is made with a bright chartreuse vegetable we call broccoflower, which is also called Romanesco broccoli. It's becoming more available at upscale supermarkets and specialty produce markets, but plain old snowy white cauliflower works (and tastes) just fine. The combination of sweet raisins and crunchy pine nuts elevate this simple dish to elegance.

Makes 6 to 8 servings.

1½-pound head cauliflower
¼ cup olive oil, divided
2 cloves garlic, minced
¼ cup raisins
½ cup vegetable stock or broth
3 tablespoons pine nuts
2 tablespoons fresh parsley, chopped
Salt and pepper to taste

1. Discard leaves and core from cauliflower, and cut into 1-inch florets. Transfer cauliflower to the slow cooker.

2. Heat 2 tablespoons oil in a small skillet over medium-high heat. Add garlic, and cook for 30 seconds, or until fragrant. Scrape garlic into the slow cooker, add raisins and stock, and stir well. Cook on Low for 4 to 6 hours or on High for 2 to 3 hours, or until cauliflower is tender.

3. While cauliflower cooks, heat remaining oil in the skillet over medium heat. Add pine nuts, and cook for 2 minutes, or until brown. Set aside.

4. Remove cauliflower from the slow cooker with a slotted spoon, and toss with pine nuts and parsley. Season to taste with salt and pepper.

> Toast small nuts and seeds, such as pine nuts, sesame seeds, and slivered almonds, in a small dry skillet over medium-high heat. Toast larger nuts such as pecans, walnuts, or whole almonds, in the oven.

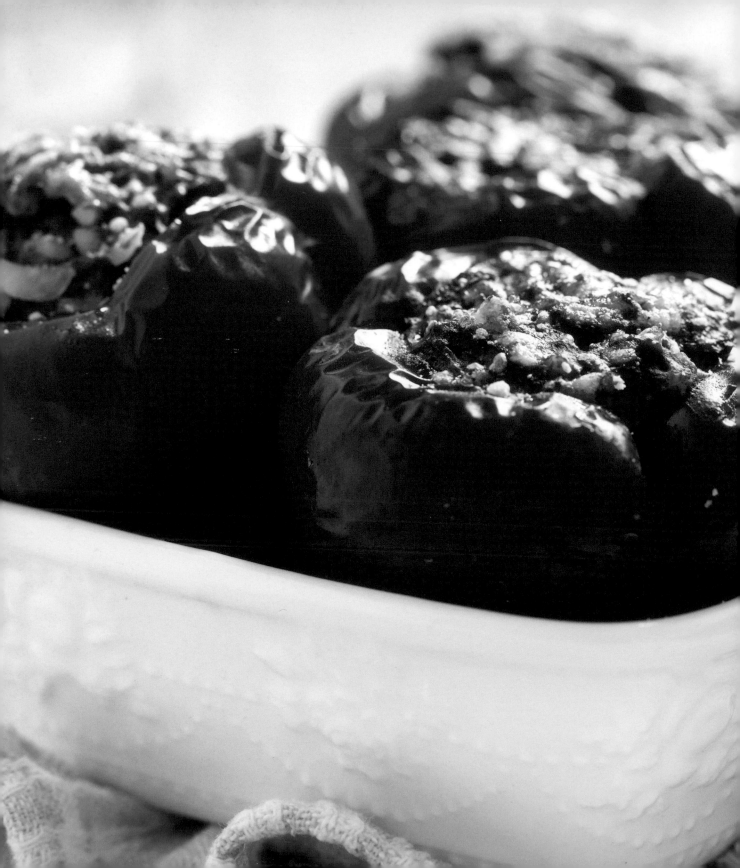

Stuffed Peppers

Make this meal as good to look at as it is to eat by using different colored bell peppers.

Makes 4 servings.

2 orange bell peppers

2 red bell peppers

2 tablespoons olive oil

3 cloves garlic, minced

1 onion, chopped

1 pound ground turkey

2 green bell peppers, seeded and chopped

1 cup diced fennel

1 cup sliced domestic mushrooms

2 tablespoons chili powder

½ teaspoon cinnamon

1 teaspoon salt

28-oz can diced tomatoes

6-oz can tomato paste

1. Working carefully, cut off the tops of the orange and red peppers and remove the seeds from inside. Set aside.

2. In a large skillet over medium-high heat, add the olive oil, onions, and garlic. Cook until onions are translucent, about 3 minutes. Add the ground chicken to the skillet and continue to cook, stirring, until meat is browned, about 5 minutes.

3. Next add the chopped green peppers, fennel, mushrooms, chili powder, salt, and cinnamon, and continue cooking, stirring constantly, until combined and heated through, about 5 minutes. Sprinkle with salt.

4. Fill the emptied peppers with the meat mixture, and place the peppers, bottoms down, into the slow cooker one at a time. In a small bowl, combine the diced tomatoes and tomato paste. Add the tomato sauce to the cooker. Cover and cook on Low for 5 to 6 hours or on High for 4 to 5 hours.

Variation:

To add some heat and additional flavor, replace the green bell pepper with some fresh, sliced hot peppers like jalapenos or habaneros.

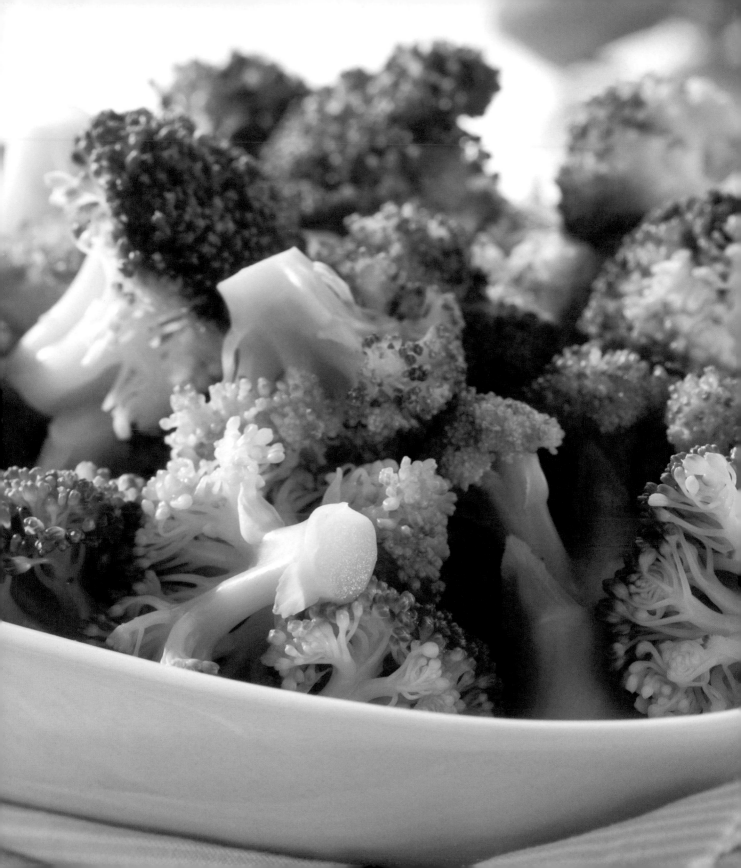

Basic Broccoli

When you want all the goodness of this delicious vegetable, here's what to do.

Makes 4 to 6 servings.

2 pounds broccoli
½ cup water
2 tablespoons olive oil
Salt and pepper to taste

1. Prepare broccoli by breaking off the florets and putting them in a colander. With the tougher stem, cut off the bottom that has the toughest part. With a sharp knife, separate the hard "skin" from the more tender center of the stem. Cut the remaining broccoli into large chunks. Rinse all the pieces in the colander and shake vigorously to remove as much water as possible.

2. Put the broccoli in the slow cooker and add that water. Drizzle with the oil, and sprinkle some salt and pepper on the broccoli. Cover and cook on Low for 2 to 3 hours or on High for 1 to 2 hours.

Variation:
Turn the tasty broccoli into an easy meal by topping with crisp-fried pancetta or bacon. Simply cut the meat into one-inch pieces, saute over medium heat to nearly crispy, remove from the pan with a slotted spoon onto a plate covered with a paper towel, and allow the crumbles to cool slightly. Add them to the broccoli and *presto*—dinner.

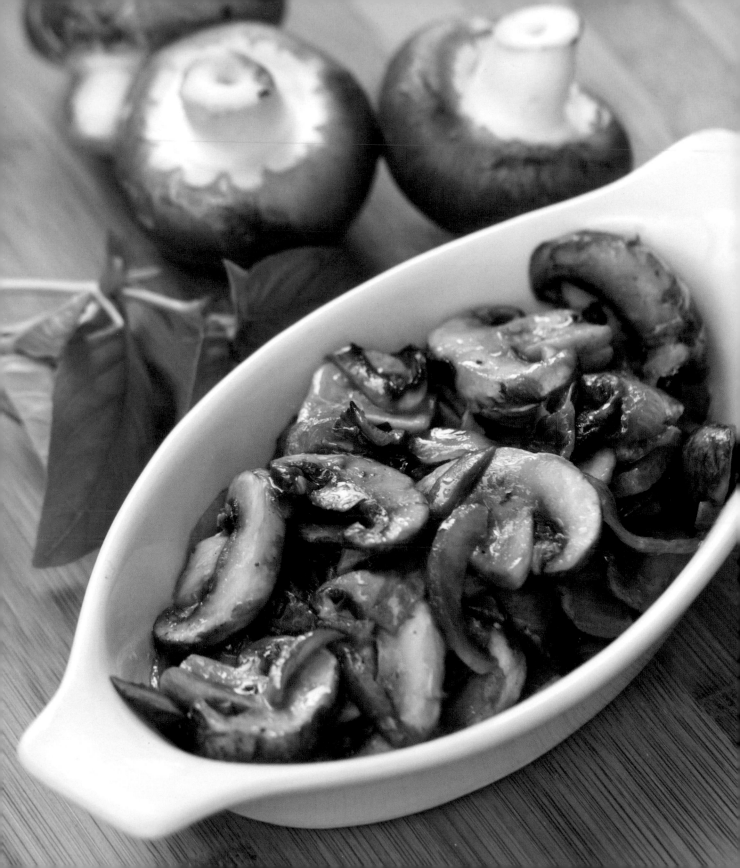

Slow and Stewy Mushrooms

Mushrooms are one of those vegetables that you can slow-cook for nearly forever so long as you keep an eye on the liquid. The longer they cook, the better they taste.

Makes 4 to 6 servings.

2 pounds mushrooms, preferably a mix of button, crimini, and Portobello

¼ cup olive oil

1 cup beef stock or broth

Salt and pepper to taste

1. Clean the mushrooms by wiping away dirt with a soft cloth or mushroom brush. Remove the toughest part of the stems, and slice into thick slices/chunks.

2. Heat the oil over medium heat in a large skillet and add the mushrooms. Stir to coat with the oil and cook, stirring for about 5 minutes.

3. Transfer the mushrooms to the slow cooker, add the beef stock, sprinkle with salt and pepper, and stir to combine. Cover and cook on Low for 7 to 9 hours, or on High for 5 to 6 hours. Stir once during cooking to be sure there is enough liquid, which there should be. For the last 30 minutes of cooking, turn to High and remove the lid. This will cook the mushroom broth down a bit to make the dish slightly thicker.

Slow-cooked mushrooms are often flavored with some vermouth during the last part of the cooking process. While there's no general consensus about the Paleo appropriateness of vermouth itself, the fact that it is made from grapes flavored with a blend of herbs, bark and roots, a dry vermouth seems to meet the requirements. Add a tablespoon to this recipe in the last 30 minutes of cooking and see what you think.

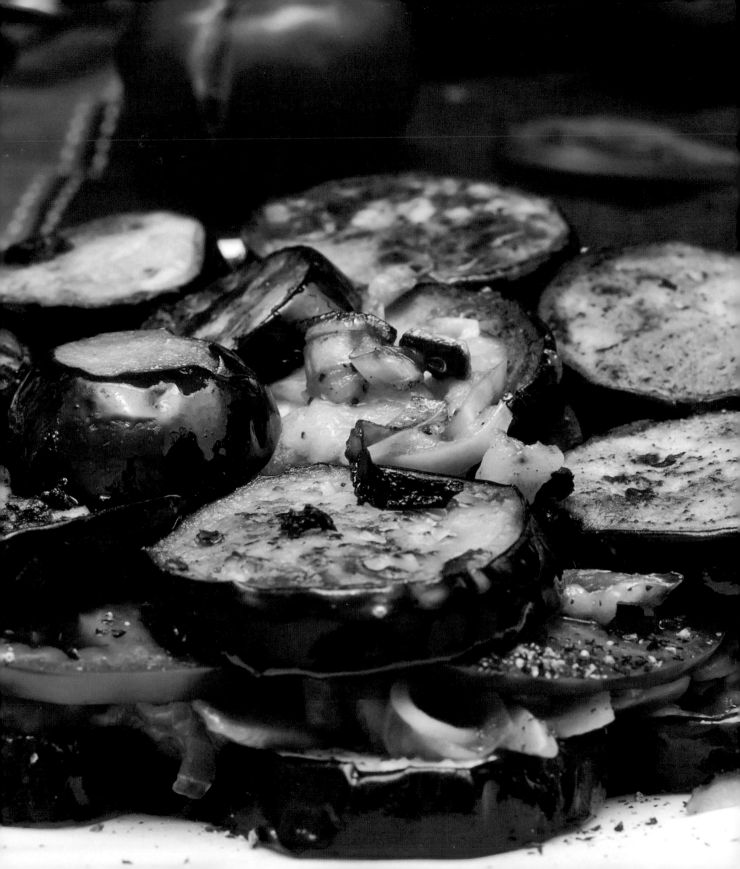

Elegant Eggplant

Layering the eggplant with the other ingredients produces an elegant casserole dish that is a sight to behold, intoxicating to sniff, and absolutely delicious!

Makes 4 to 6 servings.

2 eggplants, tops and bottoms removed, and sliced into ⅛-inch slices

8.5-oz jar sundried tomatoes packed in olive oil (see sidebar)

4 cloves garlic, sliced thin

2 to 3 tablespoons olive oil from jar of sundried tomatoes

1 tablespoon fresh rosemary needles

Salt and pepper to taste

1. Remove the sundried tomatoes from the jar, reserving the oil in the jar. Slice the tomatoes into thin strips. Drizzle a tablespoon of the oil from the sundried tomatoes on the bottom of the slow cooker.

2. Place a layer of the eggplant slices into the slow cooker, overlapping slightly to form a decorative pattern. Next, put half the sundried tomatoes on the eggplant. Then dot with half the slices of garlic.

3. Add another layer of eggplant, then tomatoes, then garlic. Finish with a layer of eggplant, then drizzle another tablespoon or two of the oil over the top. Sprinkle with rosemary.

4. Cover and cook on Low for 4 to 6 hours, or on High for 2 to 3 hours. Season with salt and pepper before serving.

> For the freshest and highest quality packaged sundried tomatoes, follow these guidelines: Check the expiration date on the package; look for tomatoes in glass jars that are packed in extra virgin olive oil (other oils are high in sodium and have an aftertaste); select 8.5-oz jars, as that is the amount you probably won't need more or less of, and so you will ensure freshness.

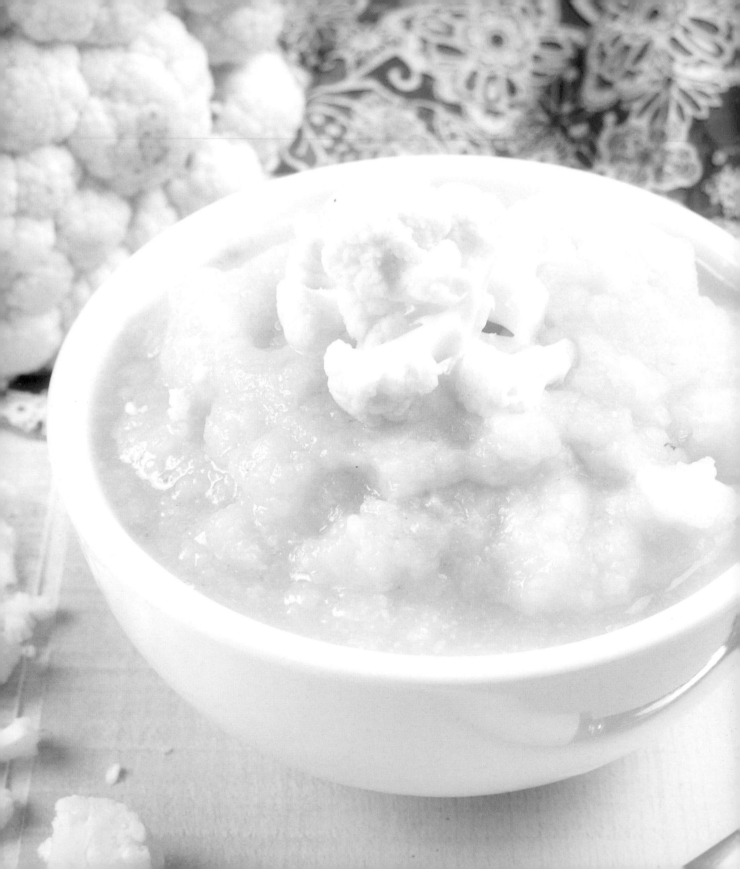

Garlic Mashed Cauliflower

This super-simple recipe produces such a flavorful and creamy dish that you will not miss traditional mashed potatoes loaded with butter or sour cream. Enjoy!

Makes 6 to 8 servings.

Two 14-oz bags of frozen cauliflower florets
Hot water to cover
1 small head of garlic, roasted
1 tablespoon coconut oil
Salt and pepper to taste

Put the cauliflower in the slow cooker and add hot tap water until the florets are just covered. Cover and cook on Low for 4 to 5 hours or on High for 2 to 3 hours until cauliflower is tender. Drain the cauliflower and put it in a bowl. Add the roasted garlic cloves and the oil, and mash with a potato masher or puree with an immersion blender, mashing to desired consistency. Season with salt and pepper.

While the cauliflower is cooking in the slow cooker, roast the garlic. To do this, preheat the oven to 400 degrees F. Peel off the outermost layers of skin on a whole clove of garlic, and cut off about ¼- to ½-inch from the top so the cloves are exposed. Put the head on a baking pan (like a muffin tin or cake pan), and drizzle about a teaspoon of olive oil on the top, being sure to coat it. Cover with aluminum foil and bake for about 30 to 40 minutes. Allow to cool before squeezing out cloves.

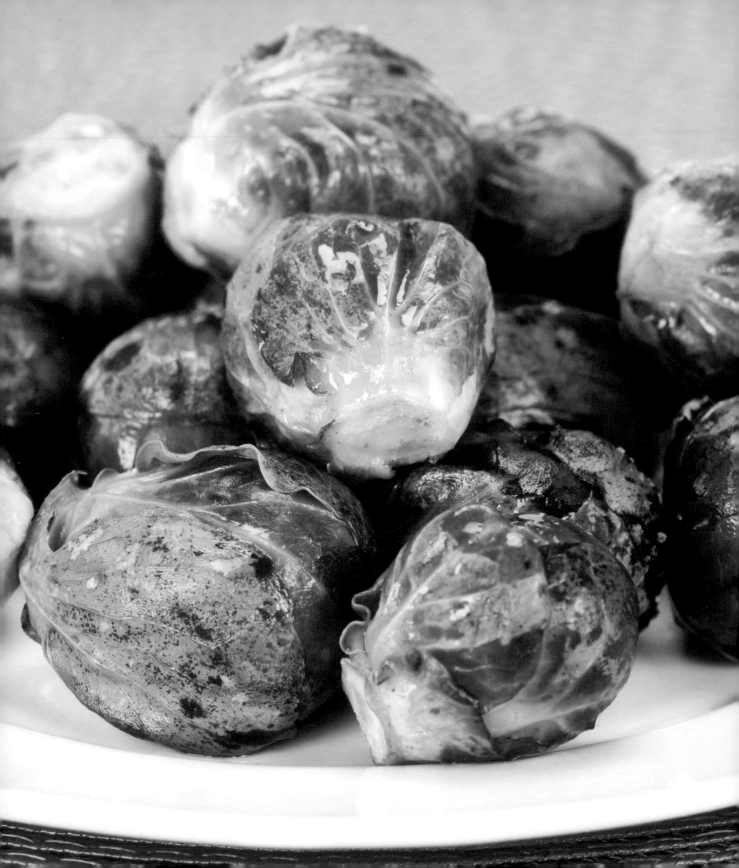

Basic Brussels Sprouts

Slow cooking this earthy veggie mellows its tanginess but brings out its woodsy depth of flavor. A touch of mustard, and seasoning with just a hint of sea salt add the perfect finish.

Makes 4 to 6 servings.

1 pound Brussels sprouts
3 tablespoons olive oil or ghee
1 teaspoon dry mustard
Pinch of sea salt

1. Wash and trim the Brussels sprouts, cutting off the coarsest part of the bottom and a layer or so of the leaves on the bottom. Cut the sprouts in half, and put them in the slow cooker.

2. In a measuring cup, mix the olive oil with the dry mustard. Pour over the Brussels sprouts. Cover and cook on Low for 3 to 4 hours or on High for 2 to 3 hours. Before serving, add a pinch of sea salt.

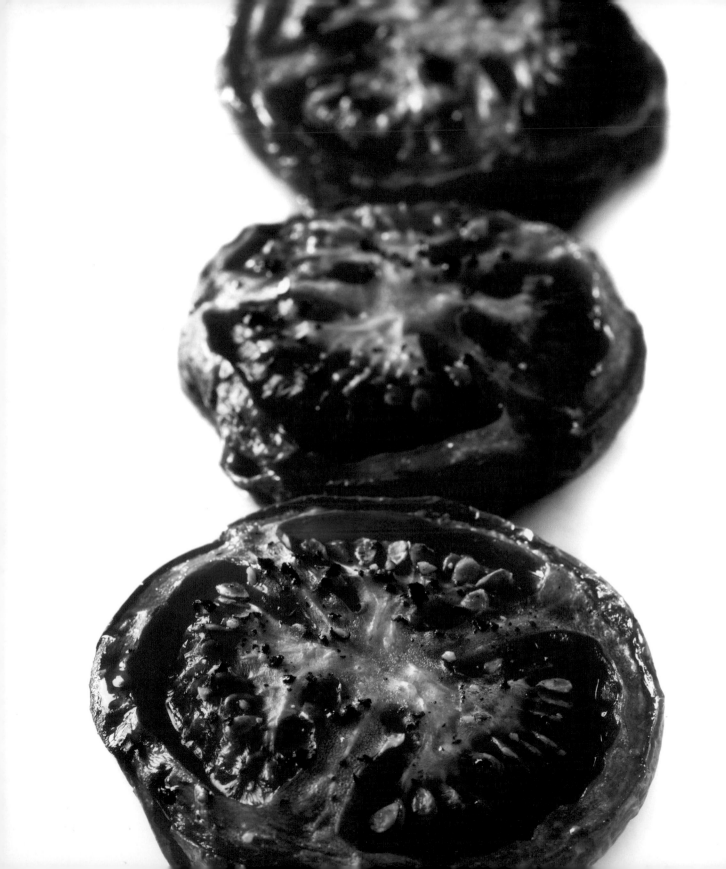

Roasted Tomatoes

Because the slow cooker retains the moisture in foods, these won't need to cook long to become moist and flavorful. Seasoned with some herbs and garlic, they make a colorful and tasty side dish.

Makes 4 to 8 servings.

4 large, ripe tomatoes, cut in half, seeds removed

2 cloves garlic, minced

1 teaspoon fresh oregano, minced, or ½ teaspoon dried

1 teaspoon fresh parsley, chopped

Salt and pepper to taste

Place cut tomatoes bottom down in the slow cooker. Sprinkle minced garlic on top, then sprinkle with the oregano. Cover and cook on Low for 3 to 4 hours or on High for 1 to 2 hours. Season with salt and pepper, and garnish with the parsley.

Summer-ripe tomatoes taste too good to cook—use them in salads, salsas, or to stuff with some meat or vegetable mix. Slow cooking is great for off-season tomatoes, preferably vine-ripened.

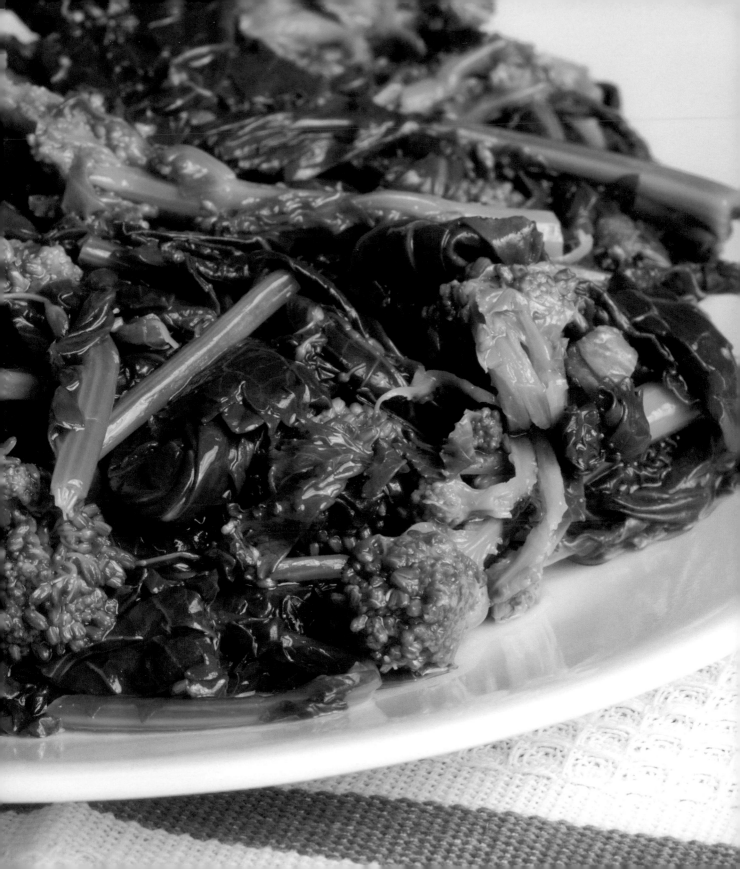

Broccoli Rabe

Consider this your "lazy" way to great broccoli rabe. Compile your ingredients, put them in the slow cooker, and come back many hours later to something truly delicious. The longer this slow cooks, the better, and if you put it on warm after 8 hours, it can go a few more hours.

Makes 4 to 6 servings.

1 pound broccoli rabe
6 large cloves garlic, sliced
1 teaspoon red pepper flakes
⅓ cup extra virgin olive oil
Salt to taste

1. Prepare the broccoli rabe by removing the tough stems and setting aside only the tops and the tender parts of the stems. Put these in a colander and rinse, then spin and/or pat dry.

2. Put the prepared broccoli rabe in the slow cooker, add the garlic, red pepper flakes, and olive oil. Cover and cook on Low for 6 to 8 hours. Do not cook on High. Season with salt to taste.

> Broccoli rabe is related to broccoli, and is a member of the turnip family. It is definitely more bitter than broccoli, and has long been popular in Italy. For an extra treat, top with toasted pignoli (pine nuts)!

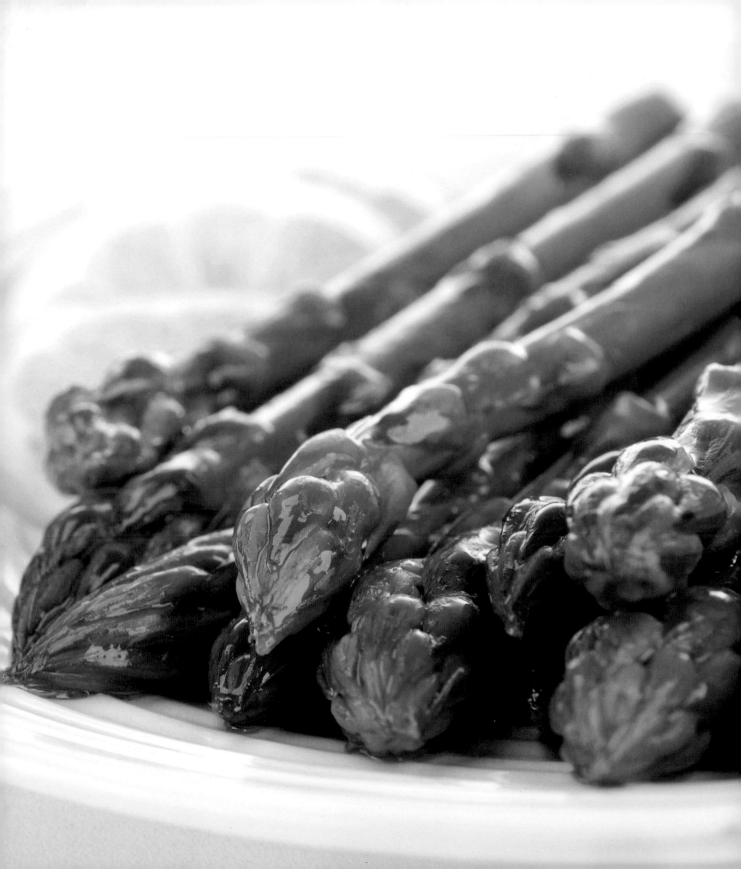

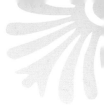

Citrusy Asparagus

Hints of lemon and orange in this dish keep the sunshine of spring in this seasonal vegetable.

Makes 4 to 6 servings.

1 seedless orange

Juice of one orange

2 tablespoons fresh-squeezed lemon juice

¼ cup olive oil

¼ red onion, minced

1 teaspoon fresh tarragon, minced

1 pound asparagus, tough parts of stems removed

Salt and pepper to taste

1. Put asparagus in the slow cooker.

2. Zest one of the oranges, then cut the white peel and pith away from the segments. Put the zest and segments in a bowl, and cut the other orange in half, squeezing its juice into the bowl.

3. Add the fresh-squeezed lemon juice, olive oil, onions, and tarragon. Pour the fruit juice mixture over the asparagus. Cover and cook on Low for 2 to 3 hours until spears are tender. Season with salt and pepper.

Variation:
You can substitute the herb lemon balm for the tarragon in this recipe. It's another of the herbs that pairs especially well with asparagus, including sage and thyme.

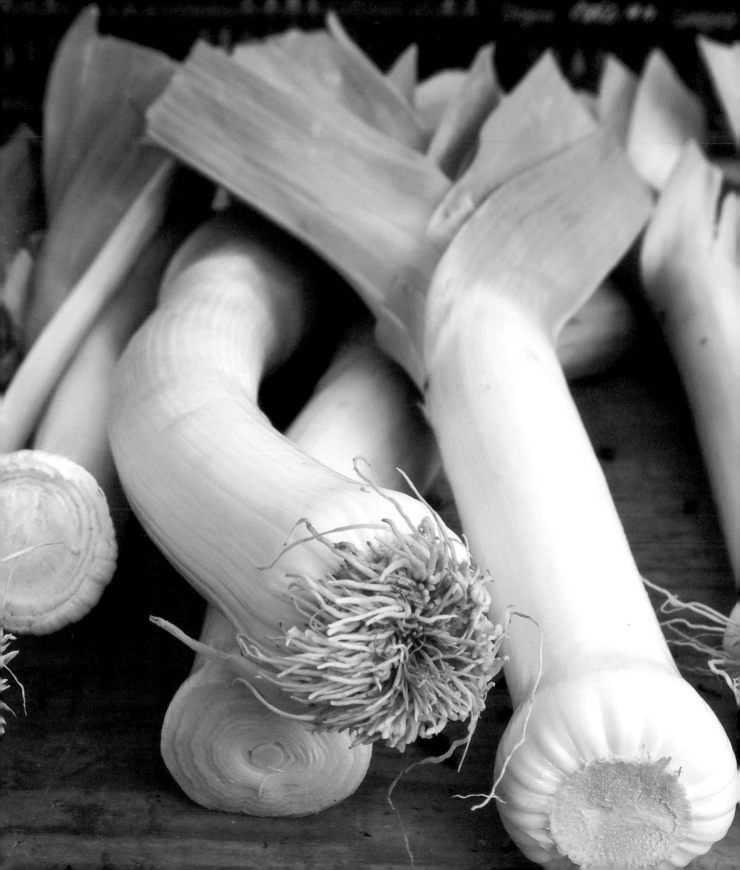

Slow-Cooked Leeks with Celery

The combination of these root vegetables with some oil and vinegar makes for a mild, delectable side dish. It's a great way to use up extras of these vegetables if you have them in your pantry.

Makes 4 to 6 servings.

4 to 6 leeks, or about 1 pound
1 head celery
3 tablespoons olive oil
3 tablespoons balsamic vinegar
Salt and pepper to taste
Fresh parsley for garnish

1. Prepare the leeks. The section that is the whitest and lightest is what you want to use, so slice off the rooted bottom, and cut off the top where the color changes from pale to darker green. Cut leeks lengthwise and rinse in cool water to be sure to remove any sand or dirt. Cut sections of leeks in half or thirds so that they fit in the slow cooker.

2. Prepare the celery. You'll want 6 to 8 stalks, with the tough bottom part and the leaves at the top trimmed off. Rinse the stalks in cool water and pat them dry. Cut celery stalks to fit in the slow cooker.

3. In a small bowl or measuring cup, combine the oil and balsamic vinegar, and whisk to combine.

4. Place stalks of celery alongside lengths of leeks in the bottom of the slow cooker. When the first layer is assembled, drizzle with the oil and vinegar, and sprinkle with salt and pepper. Continue to add layers until, drizzling and seasoning as you work up.

5. When all the celery and leeks are used up, drizzle the last of the oil and vinegar and add a final sprinkle of salt and pepper. Cover and cook on Low for about 4 hours or on High for about 2 hours. Open and flip the layers gently with a rubber spatula. Continue to cook on Low for another hour or on High for another 15 to 20 minutes. Transfer to a serving platter and garnish with fresh parsley.

The leek is a member of the onion and garlic family of Allium vegetables. It has been cultivated since ancient times, and was said to be a favorite of the Roman Emperor Nero (who reigned from 54 to 68 AD), who felt it helped with his voice. Used more extensively in Europe than the United States, the leek cooks up as a soft, fragrant onion, yielding tremendous flavor.

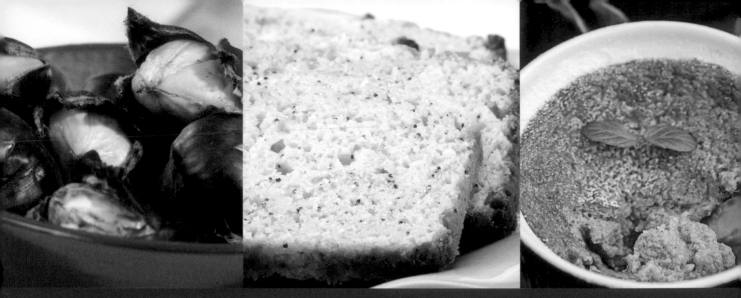

Chapter 9

Paleo *Dolci:*

A Sweet Ending Without Sugar

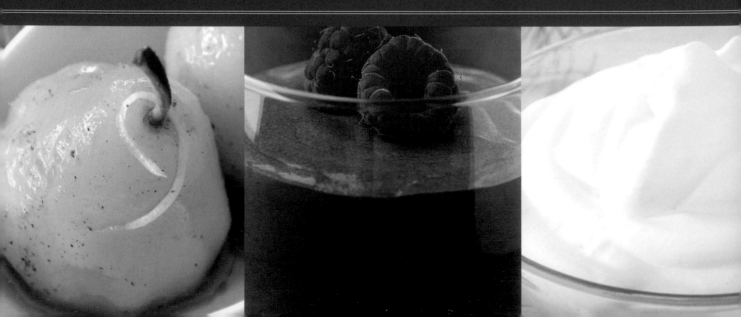

*C*lassic Italian desserts, like tiramisu or gelato, tend to be rich in cream and liqueur. While these aren't Paleo-friendly, there are other delicacies that can provide the perfect *dolci* in your day. These include chestnuts, dark chocolate, pumpkin, and of course, fruits. There's even a recipe for Paleo whipped cream here. It's not made in the slow cooker, but you can prepare it while your slow cooker is working its magic and be ready to serve it on the side.

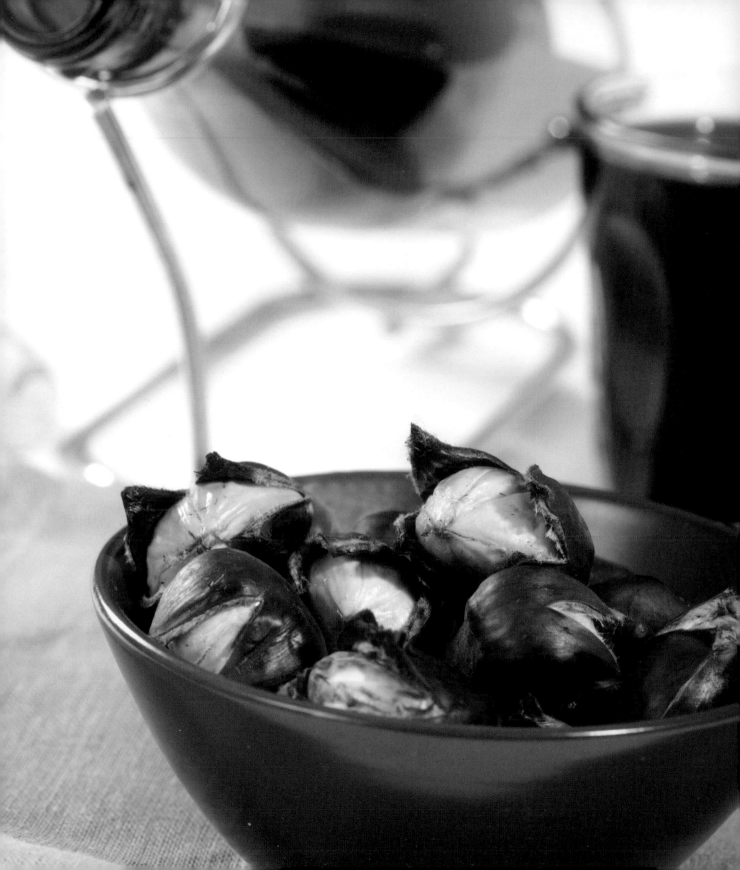

Chestnuts with Red Wine

When I saw this recipe from Marcella Hazan, I thought it would make the perfect Paleo treat. She says when she was young she would look forward to eating these wine-infused chestnuts by a roaring fire. It's easy to see why!

Makes 4 servings.

1 pound fresh large chestnuts
1 cup dry red wine
Salt
2 bay leaves

1. Prepare the chestnuts by first washing them in cold water, and then soaking them in lukewarm water for about 20 minutes. This softens the outer shell. Using a small, sharp knife, cut a slit horizontally across the middle of the chestnut, starting at the edge of a flat side and cutting across the bulging side (not the flat side). Be careful not to cut too deep, either—you don't want to penetrate the meat of the chestnut.

2. Put the slit chestnuts in the slow cooker, and cover with the wine and bay leaves. Add a pinch of salt. Cook on Low for 4 to 6 hours or on High for 1½ to 2½ hours. The chestnuts should be tender.

3. Transfer the nuts and wine to a saucepan and cook over medium heat, simmering the wine until all but a few tablespoons remain. Put the nuts in a bowl, pour the wine over them, and serve immediately, allowing guests to peel the nuts themselves.

In Italy, there are two types of chestnuts. One is small and yields two small bulbs. The other is large and yields one larger bulb. These are called *marrones* and are the kind that should be used in this recipe. Finding fresh chestnuts can be a challenge, and you may need to order them. The sales representative can assist you in choosing the right size.

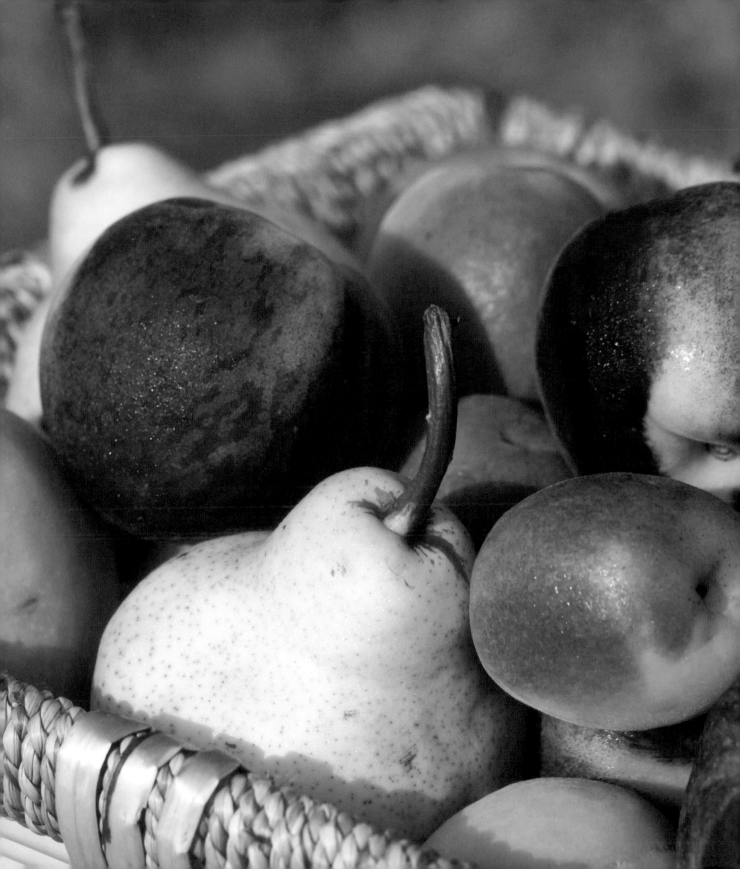

Fruit Medley

This is the perfect way to create slow-cooked, warm fruit goodness for all to enjoy.

Makes 2 to 4 servings.

1 cup pear slices

1 cup apple slices

1 cup peach slices

1 cup berries (blueberries or raspberries)

½ cup coconut crystals

¼ cup almond flour

½ teaspoon ground cinnamon

½ teaspoon ground ginger

½ teaspoon ground nutmeg

6 tablespoons coconut butter

1. Put fruit slices into the slow cooker. In a small bowl, combine coconut crystals, almond flour, and spices. Distribute evenly over fruit. Cut up butter into small pieces and sprinkle evenly over everything.

2. Cover and cook on Low for 4 to 5 hours or on High for 2 to 3 hours until fruit is soft.

> Coconut crystals are produced by dehydrating coconut sap. The sap is definitely sweet, and so raises insulin levels typical of a sugar response. But it has far less fructose than even agave, is far less processed, and contains high levels of magnesium, potassium, and B vitamins. This is why it's Paleo approved—in moderation.

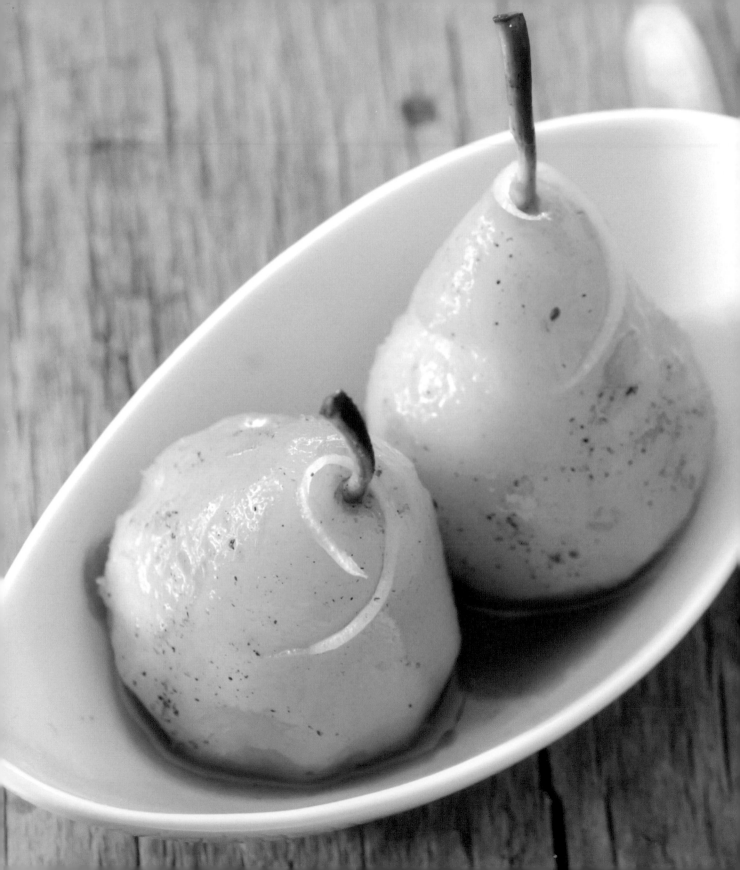

Baked Pears with Ginger

Use fully ripe pears to get the most flavor from this aromatic and satisfying dish.

Makes 4 servings.

4 large, ripe pears, cored and cut into chunks or slices

1 teaspoon ground ginger

1 teaspoon lemon zest

2 tablespoons coconut butter, cut into bits

1. Put the pear slices into the slow cooker. Sprinkle with the ginger and the lemon zest. Put bits of coconut butter over the fruit.

2. Cover and cook on Low for 3 to 4 hours or on High for about 2 hours. Serve warm or at room temperature.

Add some crunch to the recipe by topping with toasted nuts— pepitas, sesame seeds, and almonds are all good choices.

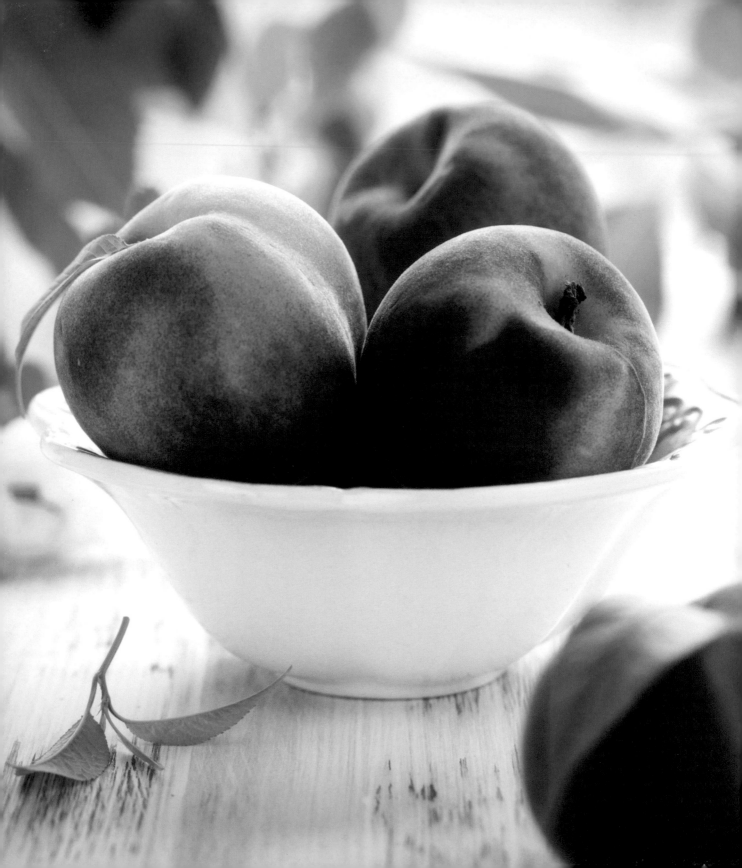

Baked Peaches

Ripe peaches are so juicy that, when slow-cooked, they make a summer slurry. Stir in some toasted nuts for added crunch when serving.

Makes 4 servings.

4 large, ripe peaches, peeled, pits removed, and cut into chunks or slices

1 teaspoon cinnamon

1 teaspoon lemon zest

2 tablespoons honey

1. Put the peach slices into the slow cooker. Sprinkle with the cinnamon and the lemon zest. Drizzle with honey.

2. Cover and cook on Low for 3 to 4 hours or on High for about 2 hours. Serve warm or at room temperature.

Variation:

Turn the recipe into a crumble or crisp by adding a topping of ½ cup almond flour mixed with 1 tablespoon coconut butter and some toasted almonds. Put the crumble on top of the fruit before cooking.

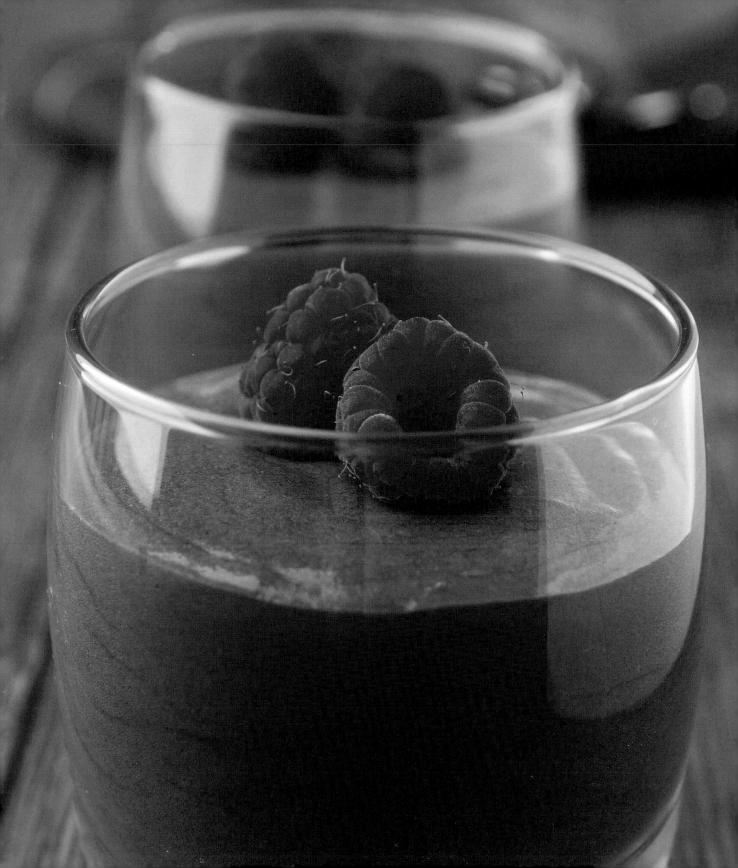

Italian Chocolate Mousse

The name of this dessert is ironic considering it's for a Paleo diet. It's not the "moose" our Paleo ancestors were savoring, that's for sure. But it's one for our modern world.

Makes 6 to 8 servings.

5 egg yolks

2 cups coconut milk

½ cup coconut crystals

1 teaspoon dark rum

1 tablespoon strong espresso coffee

¼ cup unsweetened cocoa powder

Fresh raspberries for garnish

1. Put an oven-safe casserole dish into the slow cooker. Add water around the dish so that it reaches about halfway up the side of the dish.

2. In a large bowl using a whisk, beat the egg yolks until thoroughly combined and a lighter, lemony color. Add the coconut milk, crystals, rum, espresso, and cocoa powder until well combined. Pour the mixture into the dish inside the slow cooker.

3. Cover and cook on Low for 5 to 6 hours or on High for 2 to 4 hours. The mousse should be thick but not too firm. Turn the cooker off and let the dish cool slightly in the water. Then remove it and refrigerate for an hour or longer before serving.

Variation:

Top this dish with fresh raspberries for a really elegant and decadent dessert.

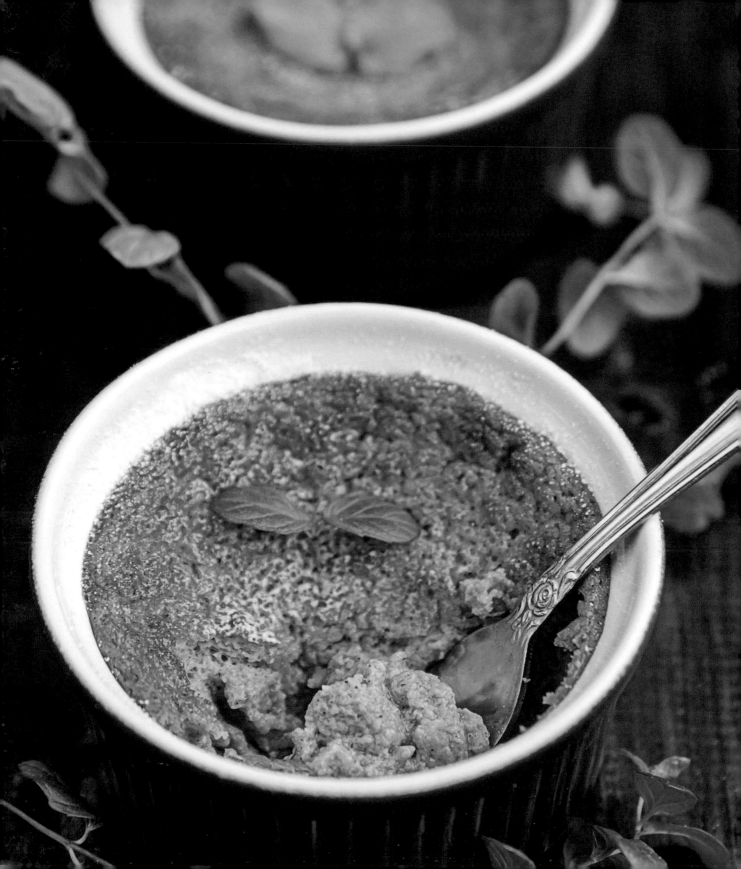

Pumpkin Custard

You can use canned organic pumpkin puree for this recipe, or you can use freshly baked or steamed pumpkin.

Makes 6 to 8 servings.

6 egg yolks

1¼ cups coconut milk

1 teaspoon pumpkin pie spice mix

½ cup coconut crystals

½ teaspoon vanilla extract

⅛ teaspoon salt

⅓ cup pumpkin puree

1. Put an oven-safe casserole dish or several ceramic ramekins into the slow cooker. Add water around the dish so that it reaches about halfway up the side of the dish(es).

2. In a large bowl using a whisk, beat the egg yolks until thoroughly combined and a lighter, lemony color. Add the coconut milk, spice mix, crystals, vanilla, and salt until well combined. Fold in the pumpkin puree. Pour the mixture into the dish inside the slow cooker.

3. Cover and cook on Low for 5 to 6 hours or on High for 2 to 4 hours. The custard should be thick but not too firm. Turn the cooker off and let the dish cool slightly in the water. Then remove it and refrigerate for an hour or longer before serving.

> **Pumpkin pie spice mix is a pre-made combination of cinnamon, ginger, nutmeg, and allspice. If you'd like to experiment with bringing out certain of these flavors, use them individually.**

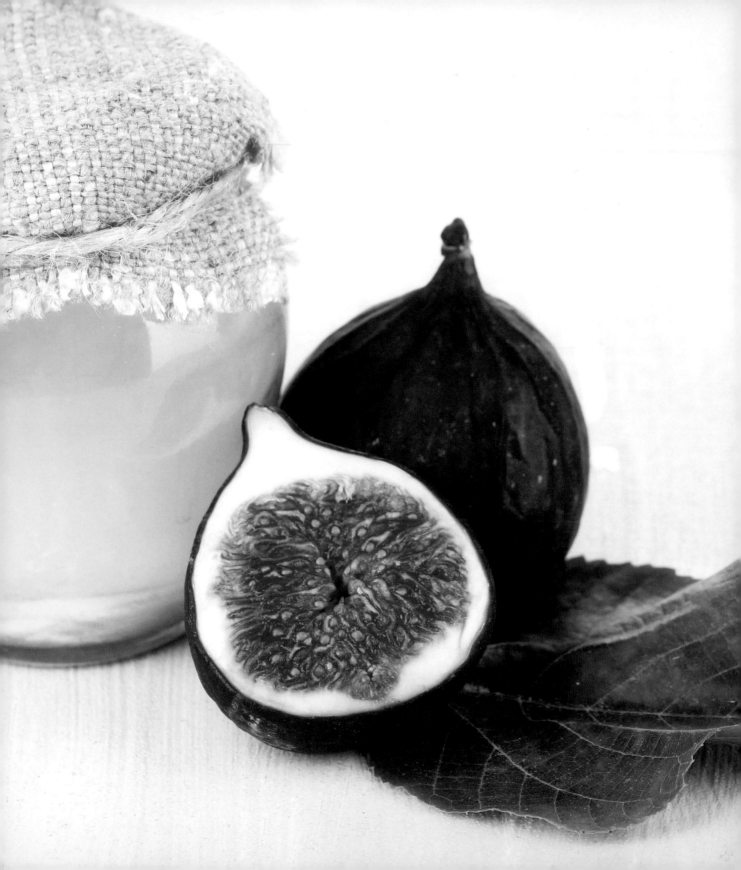

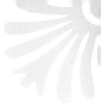

Honey-Kissed Figs

This makes a Fig Newton–like substance that has all the freshness of the figs without the additives found in the highly processed cookie centers.

Makes about 2 cups.

2 pounds fresh figs, stems removed, peeled and cut into eighths

Juice from 1 lemon

½ cup water

½ cup honey

1. Put the peeled and cut figs in the slow cooker. Squeeze the lemon over the fruit, removing the seeds that come out. Combine the water and honey in a bowl and mix. Pour over the figs.

2. Cover and cook on Low 6 to 8 hours or on High for 4 to 5 hours. Allow to cool before serving.

> Figs are actually one of the oldest known fruits, originating in northern Asia Minor—so it might have been the true treat of our Paleo ancestors. They were cooked to use as sweeteners long before the discovery of sugar. Figs are loaded with fiber, iron, and potassium.

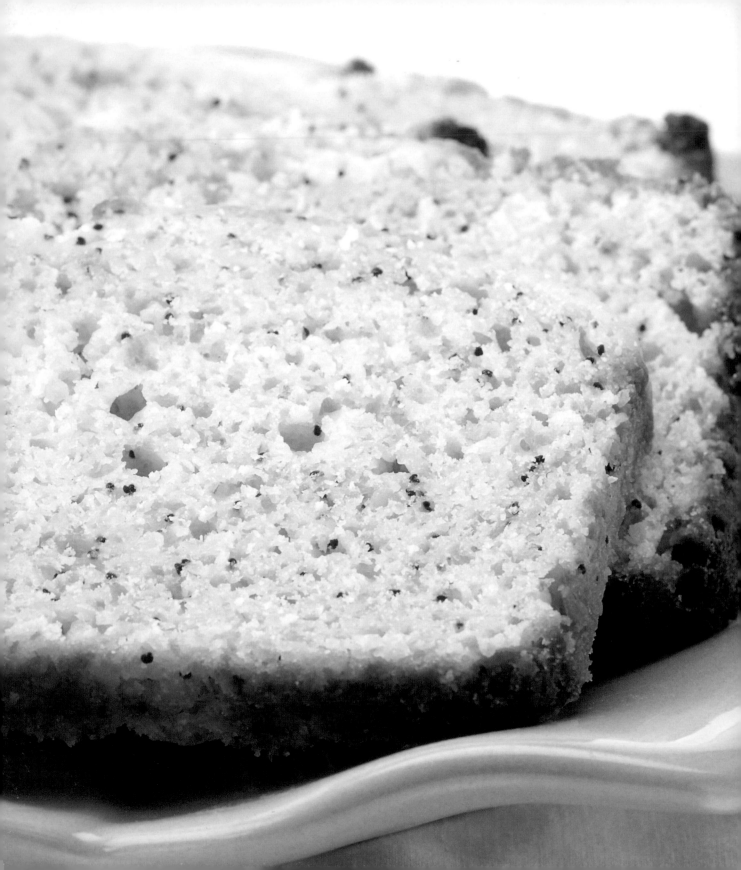

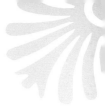

Lemon Poppy Seed Cake

Dense and lemony, this is a great dessert to satisfy your sweet tooth and your taste buds! This cake is delicious warm or chilled.

Makes 4 to 6 servings.

½ cup coconut flour

½ teaspoon salt

¼ teaspoon baking soda

6 eggs

½ cup coconut oil, melted

¼ cup honey

1 teaspoon vanilla extract

Zest of 1 lemon

2 tablespoons fresh squeezed lemon juice

1½ tablespoons poppy seeds

Fresh strawberries, blueberries, raspberries, or a combination for garnish

Non-stick cooking spray

1. Spray a bread loaf pan liberally with non-stick cooking spray and place inside the slow cooker. If it doesn't fit, line the slow cooker with aluminum foil, making sure the edges go up over the unit. Spray the aluminum foil with the non-stick cooking spray.

2. In a small bowl, combine the coconut flour, salt, and baking soda. Mix well and set aside.

3. In a large bowl, whisk the eggs until combined. Add the coconut oil, honey, vanilla, lemon zest, and lemon juice and stir to combine. Mix in the flour mixture, and then stir in the poppy seeds.

4. Pour the batter into the loaf pan or foil-lined slow cooker. Cover and cook on Low for 7 to 9 hours or on High for 4 to 5 hours. Test for doneness by inserting a toothpick in the center and seeing if it comes out clean. When cooked, remove the loaf pan from the cooker or carefully lift out the foil. Allow to cool slightly, and then transfer to a serving dish. Garnish with fresh berries if desired.

Variation:

For an even fruitier dessert, berries can be added to the batter before cooking. Use 1 cup fresh berries and fold them into the batter just before transferring to the slow cooker. You may need to increase the cooking time slightly to accommodate for the moisture of the fresh berries in the cooking process.

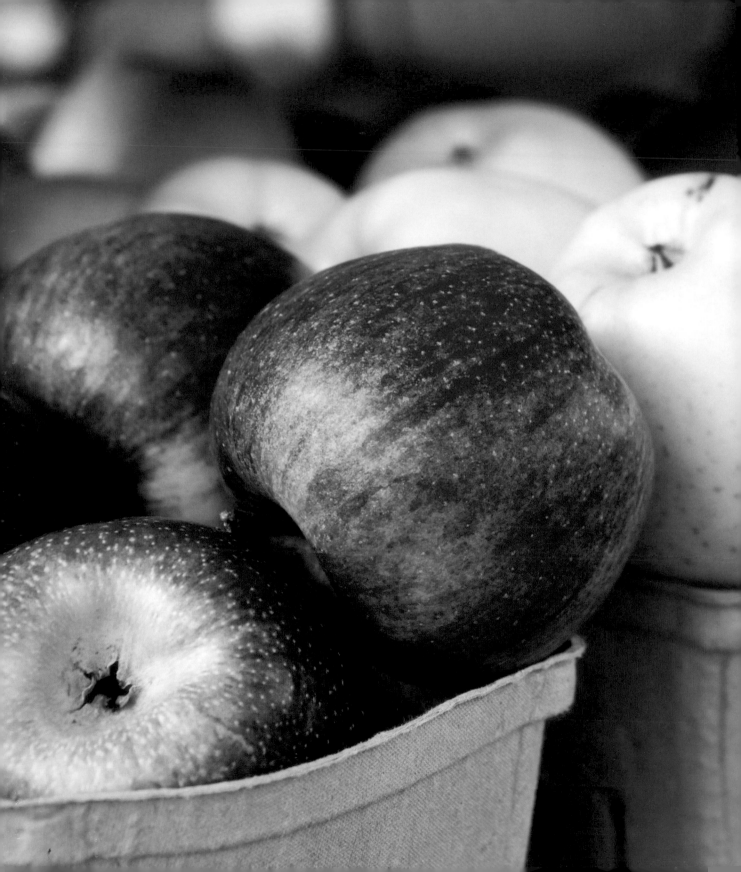

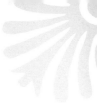

Fall Fruit Crisp

The fruits used to make this earthy dessert are available year-round in most places, so you can enjoy it any time of year.

Makes 4 to 6 servings.

3 cups baking apples, like Northern Spy or Mutsu, peeled and thinly sliced

3 cups pears, cored and cubed

½ cup dates, chopped

2 teaspoons fresh-squeezed lemon juice

1½ cups toasted pecans, crumbled

½ cup almond flour

½ teaspoon ground cinnamon

½ teaspoon ground ginger

¼ teaspoon ground nutmeg

4 tablespoons coconut butter

½ cup real maple syrup

1. In a large bowl, combine fruits, dates, and lemon juice. Mix well and transfer to the slow cooker.

2. In another bowl, combine the pecans, almond flour, spices, and maple syrup and stir to combine. Using the tines of a fork or a pastry blender, work in the coconut butter. Mixture will become a coarse "crumble." Sprinkle this evenly over the fruit mixture in the slow cooker.

3. Cover and cook on Low for 3 to 4 hours or on High for about 2 hours, or until fruit is tender. Serve warm or at room temperature.

> Maple syrup is a somewhat acceptable sweetener in the Paleo diet. While not as high-quality as honey or coconut crystals, it is relatively low in fructose and full of beneficial minerals, including manganese, potassium, iron, and calcium.

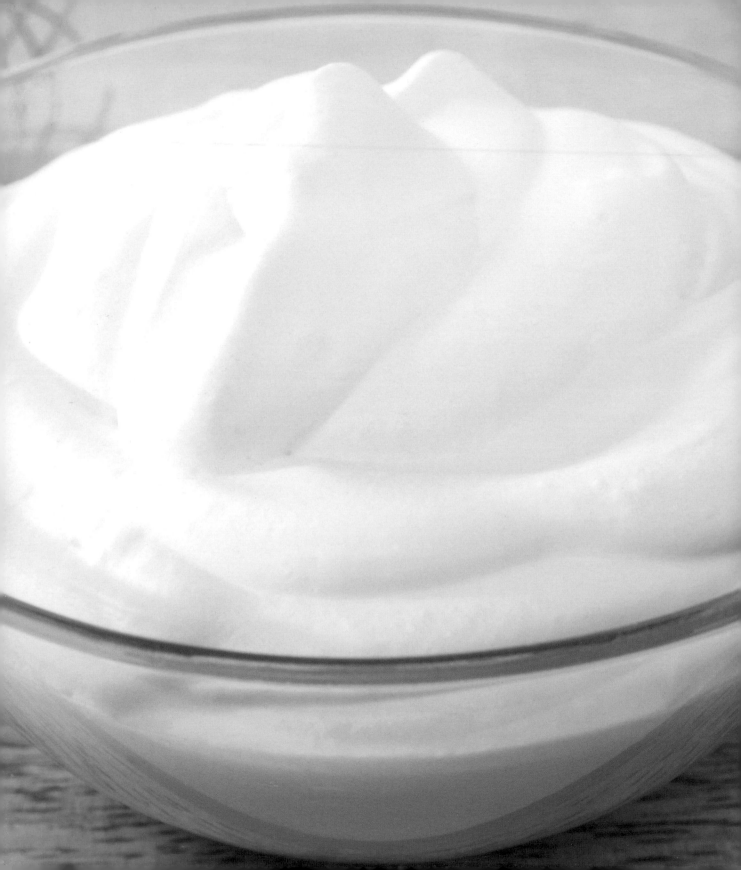

Paleo Whipped Cream

There are certain indulgences that make life really enjoyable, and fresh whipped cream is one of them. This recipe is as close as it gets to the real thing. Thank you, Jo, at Nutty Kitchen, for sharing your findings with the rest of us. I owe this one to you. Now, *mangia!*

Makes 1$^1/_2$ cups.

1 can full fat coconut milk, such as Thai Organic

Hint of vanilla, cinnamon, rum, or other flavoring

1. Put the can of coconut milk in the refrigerator overnight. Do not shake or disturb it. Let it sit. When ready, open it gently with a can opener, and scoop out the coagulated, thick milk at the top of the can. You don't want any of the water (though you can use that in other recipes or to drink).

2. Put the thick milk in a bowl, add a dash of flavoring, and beat with a mixer or a whisk until creamy. Put any leftovers in the refrigerator.

This yummy whipped cream is also a great topping for fresh fruit. You can create a really elegant dessert by serving a bowl of fresh berries topped with a dollop of the whipped coconut cream and some shavings of dark chocolate.

Paleo-Friendly Foods, A to Z

This list isn't all-inclusive, but it's a handy quick reference when you want to whip something together and you're just not sure if your ingredients are Paleo-approved. For unusual ingredients that might not be on the list, research them online. It's a great way to get involved in Paleo discussions.

Adobe Sauce
Allspice
Almonds—nuts, butter, flour, milk
Apples—all types
Apple Butter
Apple Cider Vinegar
Arrowroot Powder
Artichokes
Avocado—fruit and oil
Bacon
Baking Soda
Balsamic Vinegar
Bananas
Basil
Bay Leaf
Beef—broth/stock, whole, parts (as fresh as possible)
Beets
Blackberries
Black Pepper
Blueberries
Broccoli
Brussels Sprouts
Cabbage—all types
Capers
Carrots
Cashews—nuts and butter
Cauliflower
Cayenne Pepper
Celery
Cherries

Chicken—broth/stock, whole, parts (as fresh as possible)
Chilis—all types
Chili Powder
Chipotle
Chocolate (dark)
Chocolate Chips (dark)
Chorizo (as fresh as possible)
Cilantro—fresh and dried
Cinnamon—sticks and ground
Clementine
Cloves—whole and ground
Cocoa Powder, unsweetened
Coconut—fruit, aminos, butter, cream, flakes, flour, milk, oil (unsweetened)
Coffee
Coriander—seeds and ground
Cucumber
Cumin
Curry Powder
Dates
Dijon Mustard
Eggs—yolks and whites
Figs
Fish—all
Fish Sauce
Flaxseed—oil, meal, flour
Fruit—all
Garlic—cloves, powder, dried
Ginger—root, powder, fresh and dried
Grapes
Green Chilis
Green Onions
Green Pepper
Herbes de Provence
Honey
Hot Sauce
Italian Sausage
Italian Seasoning
Jalapenos
Kale

Lamb—chops, ribs, leg, roast, shoulder (all), fresh
Lemon—all parts, fresh
Lime—all parts, fresh
Macadamia—nuts, butter
Mango
Maple Syrup
Mushrooms—button, domestic, Portobello, crimini, shiitake, all types (fresh)
Mustard—powder, seeds
Nut Butters—all except peanut butter
Nutmeg—fresh and dried
Olive Oil
Olives—all types
Onion—yellow, white, red, pearl (all types)—fresh or frozen, unprocessed
Orange   all parts, fresh
Oregano—fresh and dried
Paprika—sweet and hot
Parsley—fresh and dried
Peach
Pecans—raw, butter
Pickles
Pineapple
Pistachios
Plantains
Poblano Pepper
Poppy Seeds
Pork—chops, ribs, bacon, sausage, offal (as fresh as possible)
Portobello Mushrooms
Protein Powder
Pumpkin—vegetable, seeds (unprocessed)
Raisins
Red Onion
Red Pepper
Red Pepper Flakes
Red Wine
Red Wine Vinegar
Rosemary—fresh and dried
Sage—fresh and dried

Salmon
Scallions
Sesame Oil
Shallots
Short Ribs
Shrimp—raw, cooked, frozen (unprocessed)
Spinach
Squash
Strawberries
Sun-dried Tomatoes
Sweet Potatoes
Tilapia
Tomato—fruit, and unseasoned canned, diced, sauce, paste
Turkey—whole, ground, pieces (unprocessed)
Unsweetened Cacao Powder
Unsweetened Coconut Flakes
Unsweetened Coconut Powder
Unsweetened Shredded Coconut
Vegetable Broth
Vegetables—all except legumes
Walnut—nuts, oil, and butter
White Wine Vinegar
Yellow Mustard
Zucchini
Vanilla—bean, extract

Index

About Cider Mill Press
Book Publishers

Good ideas ripen with time. From seed to harvest, Cider Mill Press brings fine reading, information, and entertainment together between the covers of its creatively crafted books. Our Cider Mill bears fruit twice a year, publishing a new crop of titles each spring and fall.

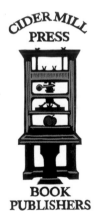

Visit us on the Web at
www.cidermillpress.com
or write to us at
12 Spring Street
PO Box 454
Kennebunkport, Maine 04046